Responding to the interests and concerns of Member countries with regard to growth in health expenditures, the OECD in 1985 published *Measuring Health Care 1960-1983,* an international comparative compendium of health care financing, expenditure, utilisation and price statistics. The Working Party on Social Policy of the Manpower and Social Affairs Committee has continued to emphasize the importance of health care financing and delivery issues, and these were one of the principal topics at a Joint Japanese/OECD Conference of High-Level Experts held in Tokyo in November 1985. *Health and Pension Policies Under Economic and Demographic Constraints,* published in 1987, contains a series of papers on various aspects of health care financing and delivery prepared for this Conference by international experts.

This study, prepared by George J. Schieber of the Directorate for Social Affairs, Manpower and Education, contains an extensive analysis of health care financing and delivery trends, issues and policies in OECD countries. It is published on the responsibility of the Secretary General.

Also available

"OECD: Social Policy Studies" Series

No. 3. LIVING CONDITIONS IN OECD COUNTRIES. A Compendium of Social Indicators (February 1986)
(81 85 04 1) ISBN 92-64-12734-8   166 pages   £6.50   US$13.00   F65.00   DM29.00

No. 2. MEASURING HEALTH CARE 1960-1983. Expenditure, Costs and Performance (November 1985)
(81 85 06 1) ISBN 92-64-12736-4   162 pages   £9.00   US$18.00   F90.00   DM40.00

No. 1. SOCIAL EXPENDITURE 1960-1990. Problems of Growth and Control (March 1985)
(81 85 01 1) ISBN 92-64-12656-2   98 pages   £7.50   US$15.00   F75.00   DM33.00

EMPLOYMENT GROWTH AND STRUCTURAL CHANGE (February 1985)
(81 85 02 1) ISBN 92-64-12659-7   226 pages   £9.50   US$19.00   F95.00   DM42.00

THE WELFARE STATE IN CRISIS (September 1981)
(81 81 01 1) ISBN 92-64-12192-7   274 pages   £7.00   US$17.50   F70.00   DM35.00

To be Published

HEALTH AND PENSION POLICIES UNDER ECONOMIC AND DEMOGRAPHIC CONSTRAINTS

Prices charged at the OECD Bookshop.

*THE OECD CATALOGUE OF PUBLICATIONS and supplements will be sent free of charge
on request addressed either to OECD Publications Service, Sales and Distribution Division,
2, rue André-Pascal, 75775 PARIS CEDEX 16, or to the OECD Sales Agent in your country.*

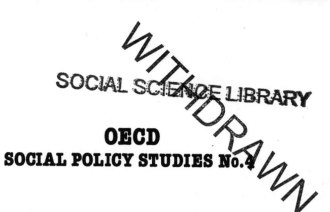

OECD
SOCIAL POLICY STUDIES No. 4

FINANCING AND DELIVERING HEALTH CARE

A Comparative Analysis
of OECD Countries

ORGANISATION FOR ECONOMIC CO-OPERATION AND DEVELOPMENT

Publié en français sous le titre :

LA SANTÉ :
FINANCEMENT ET PRESTATIONS
Analyse comparée des pays de l'OCDE

TABLE OF CONTENTS

LIST OF TABLES

LIST OF CHARTS

FOREWORD

Health care expenditure is the second largest social expenditure item in OECD countries and currently accounts for over 7 per cent of GDP. Health services account for over 9 per cent of total public and private final consumption expenditures and for almost 5 per cent of total employment. Over the past twenty years real health spending has increased substantially faster than real GDP. Much of this growth has been due to the increased demand for services and the expansion of health care delivery systems engendered by the growth in public and private financing programmes and the concomitant increasing sophistication of modern medicine. Future demographic changes combined with new technological developments could pose significant additional financing burdens on both public and private health insurance systems.

Health systems embody the social, economic and cultural imprints of different societies. They embody the often competing, often complementary objectives of numerous public and private organisations and individuals. Despite these diversities, all countries attempt to provide access to necessary, high-quality care for their citizens, while achieving efficient production of medically-effective services.

Over the past decade the ability of societies to achieve these potentially conflicting objectives has been called into question. Health financing and delivery systems that were initially conceived to provide access to services appeared to be less successful at achieving efficiency. Governments and private purchasers began to question the cost- and health-effectiveness of the additional services they were purchasing. With the achievement of almost universal access in most countries, efficiency and effectiveness issues have moved to the forefront of the policy debate.

The principal problem in designing policies to achieve efficiency stems from the difficulties in defining and measuring the output of health systems, as well as the general lack of clinically agreed-upon standards of appropriateness of medical care. Compounding the problems of measuring health outcomes and appropriateness of medical care is the interaction of individuals' health status with almost all other social and economic aspects of society. Nutrition, stress, sedentary lifestyles, alcohol and tobacco consumption, and numerous other environmental and social factors, such as unemployment, all affect an individual's health status. The importance of societally-induced illness is central to the health care financing debate. Similarly, changing demographic structures resulting from low birth rates, divorce, increased female labour force participation and population ageing necessitate placing an increased emphasis on the interaction between health, pensions, housing and other social assistance programmes. Clearly the policy debate on health care financing and delivery must extend well beyond the purview of the health programmes themselves.

The current debate also involves difficult moral and ethical issues. Many of the current advances in molecular biology and genetic engineering raise controversial ethical questions. Decisions to withhold or discontinue life-sustaining technologies, whether based on individual preferences or other considerations, also raise difficult moral questions.

This volume attempts to provide a framework for understanding the complex medical, social and economic forces underlying health care financing and delivery systems. It provides a background for the policy debate underway in all countries. Hopefully, it will contribute to the development of effective policies that will consolidate past gains and accommodate future changes.

Chapter 1

INTRODUCTION AND SUMMARY

Introduction

This report analyses health care expenditure, price, and utilisation trends in OECD countries. In 1984 the 780 million citizens of the 24 OECD countries consumed over $800 billion worth of health services, more than $1 000 per person. On average almost 80 per cent of all health expenditures are financed by the public sector. Health care expenditures are the second largest social expenditure item in the OECD, accounting for almost 15 per cent of all public spending, and 25 per cent of all social spending. Public expenditures on health account for almost 6 per cent of GDP, while overall health expenditures are approaching 8 per cent. The health industry is generally one of the largest employers in all OECD countries, and in several countries medical goods and services are a significant element in their international trade.

Over the past twenty years health expenditures have increased substantially faster than overall economic growth, resulting in increasing proportions of social resources being devoted to the health sector. Much of this growth has resulted from certain unique structural characteristics that cause external diseconomies and market failure in the production and consumption of health care. Given progress in medical technologies, future demographic change, and potential future financing constraints, governments are increasingly concerned about their ability to provide universal access to necessary services. Difficult financial and ethical questions concerning the reconciliation of needs and costs, the rationing of care, and choices between therapy and death are at the forefront of the policy agendas in all OECD countries.

Table 1 provides aggregate information on the macro-economic importance of the health sector in each of the OECD countries by displaying the share of public and total health expenditures in GDP, the share of (public and private) health consumption in total (public and private) final consumption expenditure, and health care employment as a proportion of total employment.

For the OECD area as a whole public health care expenditures in 1984 averaged 5.6 per cent of GDP,

ranging from 3.6 per cent in Greece to 8.6 per cent in Sweden. Overall health spending averaged 7.2 per cent of GDP, ranging from 4.6 in Greece to 10.7 in the United States. Health expenditures are also a significant part of total final consumption expenditure (TCE), averaging over 9 per cent of TCE in the OECD, from a low of 5.3 per cent in Greece to a high of 11.6 in the United States.

The health care sector is also one of the largest employers. On average the health care sector accounts for almost 5 per cent of all employment, ranging from a low of 2.1 per cent in Greece to a high of 7.8 per cent in Sweden.

While the health sector is important in terms of its aggregate impact, it has proven to be one of the least

Table 1

SIZE OF HEALTH SECTOR, 1984

	Public Health to GDP	Total Health to GDP	Health Consumption to TCE	Health Employment to Total Employment
	(Percent)			
Australia	6.6	7.8	9.1	6.9 (83)
Austria	4.4	7.2	9.5 (83)	5.4 (82)
Belgium	5.7	6.2	-	4.5 (81)
Canada	6.2	8.4	-	4.8 (81)
Denmark	5.3	6.3	7.8 (81)	4.8 (80)
Finland	5.4	6.6	7.8	5.9 (82)
France	6.5	9.1	11.0 (82)	4.4 (83)
Germany	6.4	8.1	10.0	2.2 (80)
Greece	3.6	4.6	5.3	2.1 (81)
Iceland	6.5	7.9	8.3 (80)	-
Ireland	6.9	8.0	9.8 (83)***	5.2 (83)
Italy	6.1	7.2	8.5 (82)	2.6 (83)
Japan	4.8	6.6	9.2	2.9 (81)
Luxembourg	-	6.4 (82)	-	-
Netherlands	6.8	8.6	-	7.2 (84)
New Zealand	4.4	5.6	-	5.7 (80)
Norway	5.6	6.3	9.6	10.3*(84)
Portugal	3.9	5.5	-	2.5 (82)
Spain	4.2	5.8	-	3.3 (83)
Sweden	8.6	9.4	10.7 (83)	7.8 (83)
Switzerland	-	7.8 (82)	10.7 ***	5.6 (82)
Turkey	-	-	-	-
United Kingdom	5.3	5.9	6.8 ***	5.3 (83)
United States	4.4	10.7	11.6 (83)	5.3 (83)
Average	5.6	7.2	9.1	4.7**

Notes: TCE - Total (public and private) final consumption expenditure.
  *   - Includes part-time as well as full-time (e.g. figures not in full-time equivalents), and a large number of those employed in social services.
  ** - Excludes Norway. The average is 5.0 per cent if Norway is included.
  *** - Based on OECD National Accounts data supplemented by other National sources.

Sources: Measuring Health Care 1960-1983, OECD, Paris, 1985. Figures for 1984 are estimates based on the same source documents and method. National Accounts, Volumes I-II, OECD, Paris, 1986.

controllable and least understood sectors, for a variety of historical, political, economic and socio-medical reasons. Prior to the 1930s there were relatively few efficacious medical interventions, so that the main improvements in life expectancy were due to improved standards of sanitation and living. Deaths from infectious and parasitic diseases, the principal causes of death, were radically reduced as a result of these factors. Expensive institutional therapies and sophisticated medical technologies to treat most illnesses were virtually non-existent. Effective medical interventions began to appear only in the 1930s, and became widely available in the late 1940s and 1950s. In the post-war prosperity of the 1950s and 1960s OECD countries expanded their health care financing and delivery systems. In the context of social solidarity, the welfare state, and the great society, universal access to health care, generally publicly financed, was seen as a right for all citizens. In the 1950s, 1960s and early 1970s health care systems expanded rapidly, as public and private financing supported and helped create new effective demand and delivery system capacity.

However, beginning in the 1970s and continuing into the 1980s, the recessions in most OECD countries engendered by the oil shocks, coupled with rapid increases in health care expenditures, put governments under strong financial pressures. Governments raised serious questions concerning the cost at which access to care and delivery system capacity had been achieved; whether the public purse could continue to afford new and expensive technologies in the context of future demographic changes and slower economic growth; and what had been and would be the marginal benefits of additional expenditures.

It has become increasingly clear that health care financing and delivery systems that were initially designed to assure access and promote the capacity of delivery systems were not well suited to the achievement of efficiency in either the provision or the use of services. Indeed there is a near-universal consensus that there are substantial allocational inefficiencies in the provision and use of health services, and that there is substantial excess capacity in terms both of manpower and facilities. As a result, much of the focus on health policy has shifted from access to cost control.

Much of the rationale for public intervention to assure access, as well as the difficulties in assuring efficiency, stem from the inherent characteristics of health care. Many of these stem from the basic nature of the commodity itself (e.g. unpredictability of needs, imperfect knowledge on the part of the consumer, barriers to entry for suppliers, etc.), while others stem from the interaction of these endogenous characteristics with exogenous features of financing, insurance, and delivery systems. The result is almost invariably allocational and distributional inefficiencies in demand and supply in virtually all health systems. Examples include: distributions of illness unrelated to ability to pay; the bulk of expenditure being concentrated on a relatively small proportion of the population with high medical care needs; consumer dependence on the decisions of medical care providers who frequently have a financial stake in the outcome of the decision; medical ethics and consumer demands which tend to support additional resource use to prolong life irrespective of patient prognosis and costs; benefit and cost-sharing structures which frequently provide incentives for the provision of costly institutional over ambulatory care; tax structures which provide incentives for over-insuring; perverse reimbursement and service delivery mechanisms which provide few incentives for the cost-effective provision of services; lack of cost-consciousness on the part of the consumer at the point of service delivery; premature implementation of costly new medical technologies without proper evaluation; lack of mechanisms to eliminate costly duplications of facilities; and an inability to deal with a growing supply of physicians and other health care resources in conjunction with continued maldistribution by location and specialty.

There is also a growing awareness that much illness is societally-induced, due to lifestyles and environmental factors. Preventing or reducing such diseases of civilisation is difficult because it involves fundamental changes in individual and societal values and behaviour. Economic incentives to change such behaviour are often marginally effective at best, and government policies to enforce behaviour change must often balance individual freedom against perceived increased government interference.

There is also significant evidence that social functioning, health and well-being can be seriously affected by job insecurity, underemployment and unemployment. Both macro and micro economic evidence indicate that the unemployed and their families suffer additional morbidity and mortality from changes in body chemistry that lead to increases in blood pressure, heart disease, mental illness and suicides[1].

Moreover, increased life expectancy achieved as a result of improved standards of living and health systems, combined with expected future demographic developments, are changing much of the emphasis of health financing and delivery systems from acute to chronic care. The integration of acute and long-term care financing and delivery systems, the focus on social as well as medical services, issues of family as compared with societal responsibilities, and difficult ethical choices between further treatment and death are concerns faced by all OECD countries.

A further important issue is the present inability to measure the effects of health expenditures in achieving their intended purpose, the assurance of "good health". Indeed this is the crux of the present problem. There is no single generally-accepted and empirically valid measure of "good health". Hence, there is little information relating increases in health expenditures to improvements in health. Furthermore, the development of outcome measures is only at a preliminary stage.

This report analyses and compares the health systems

of OECD countries, estimates the future impact of demographic change on expenditures, and reviews the policy options to assure access, quality and efficiency under present and future economic constraints. The report is in nine sections. Chapter 2 contains a detailed discussion of the inherent problems in making international comparisons, and provides detailed comparative information on international differences in age structures, medical practice patterns, price levels, and the concentration of expenditures. Chapter 3 discusses the structural features and implicit incentives of the health care financing and delivery systems of OECD countries in terms of financing procedures, eligibility criteria, benefits provided, reimbursement procedures, and organisation and development of the delivery system. Chapter 4 discusses the problems of measuring the effectiveness of health expenditures, and provides comparative information on mortality, morbidity, and costs of illness. In Chapter 5 the growth in total and public health expenditures since 1960 is analysed. The composition of health expenditures in terms of institutional, ambulatory, pharmaceutical, and other care is discussed, and underlying differences in prices and utilisation of hospital and physician services are analysed in Chapter 6. Chapter 7 analyses the factors responsible for differences in health expenditures across countries. In Chapter 8, potential impacts of future demographic and technological changes are considered, and their resulting effects on the demand for, and financing and delivery of, long-term care are analysed. In Chapter 9, the underlying difficulties in policy formulation are summarised, a taxonomy of policy options is provided, and recent actions undertaken by OECD countries are examined.

Summary of Main Findings

The principal findings of the report, based on analyses of epidemiologic, demographic, and economic information, indicate:

- Changes in the incidence of morbidity towards chronic diseases;
- Significant improvements in life expectancy and infant mortality in all countries, but nevertheless with significant remaining differences among countries;
- Until quite recently, real growth in health expenditures well in excess of real GDP growth, posing potential future problems for governments if slower growth persists;
- Concentration of health expenditures on a relatively small proportion of the population with high medical care needs;
- Awareness that increased utilisation and intensity of services is the principal endogenous factor driving health care expenditures;
- Large increases in the number of hospital beds and physicians, so that most countries, despite

some regional and specialty shortages, generally face significant surpluses of both;
- Significant differences, not only across but also within countries, in availability and use of resources both in terms of hospital stays and surgical rates, which do not appear to be related to health outcomes;
- Substantial increases in hospital expenditures, large differences among countries in per capita, per admission, per bed, and per day expenditures, growth of hospital prices generally in excess of the overall inflation rate, and hospitals representing an increasingly larger share of total health expenditures;
- Evidence of inappropriate use of services, resulting in misallocations of resources and adverse iatrogenic effects;
- Demonstrated cost-saving potential of prospective payment systems, competitive bidding arrangements, and capitated reimbursement arrangements, as well as new types of delivery arrangements such as ambulatory surgery centres, birthing clinics, and hospices;
- Large capital and operating costs associated with the implementation of certain new technologies, necessitating planning from both cost and quality perspectives;
- Significant differences in physician incomes across countries, general perceptions, backed by some evidence, that relative fee imbalances contribute to inefficiency, and realisation of the importance of the physician's central decision-maker role;
- Programmes concentrating on health promotion, health education, and lifestyles as effective means of reducing health spending;
- Increased consciousness of the amount of resources devoted to certain population groups, including terminally ill patients, and to decisions by individuals concerning the right to die;
- Continued concerns about underutilisation of services by certain population subgroups, despite almost universal access;
- Increased concern about the financing and delivery of long-term care services, the interaction between health and social service systems, and the importance of appropriate case management;
- Mixed philosophical views about cost-sharing, despite growing behavioural evidence about its effects on reducing utilisation and its relatively small negative effects on health outcomes.

The difficulties in measuring health outcomes, appropriateness of medical care, efficiency, and distributional objectives, as well as the concomitant lack of generalisable behavioural studies of reimbursement, delivery systems organisation, and supply response, mean that there is an insufficiently solid basis for making strong policy recommendations – other than to improve the quality of data and studies concerning the measurement of the key aspects of health care. However, policy has to be made, even in the absence of adequate information. It would appear, on the basis of the limited amount of evidence available, that various approaches, some market-oriented including competitive bidding, new delivery arrangements such as Health Maintenance Organisations (HMOs), and prospective reimbursement systems, others regulatory, such as tight limits on hospital beds and equipment, are effective mechanisms for inducing more efficient use of resources[2]. Moreover, individuals and societies have begun to recognise the concept of limits and the difficult economic, social and ethical choices that such limits impose.

NOTES AND REFERENCES

1. See *Health Policy Implications of Unemployment*, World Health Organisation, Regional Office for Europe, Copenhagen, 1985.
2. Much of the competition versus regulation debate is a question of semantics. Furthermore, competition and regulation cannot be discussed in isolation. The real policy issues involve managed or regulated competition. See Alain C. Enthoven, "Managed Competition in Health Care and the Unfinished Agenda", *Health Care Financing Review*, Annual Supplement, 1986.

Chapter 2

ISSUES IN INTERNATIONAL COMPARISONS

This chapter describes a number of basic problems in making international comparisons, and provides descriptive information on several of the demographic, economic and medical practice factors that can account for differences in health expenditures. International comparisons are difficult to make, because of the limited comparability of data and methodological problems arising from comparing different economic, demographic, cultural and institutional structures. In addition to well-documented data problems, another series of difficulties in performing cross-country comparisons deals with the appropriate indices of comparability.

Comparability of data is a significant, albeit frequently neglected, problem in the making of international comparisons. There are no universally accepted "social accounts" definitions of health aggregates or disaggregates. Boundaries of health systems differ (e.g. social services, school health, environmental health, etc.), and there are no universally accepted definitions of "hospitals", "nursing homes", etc. Although many of the data analysed here are based on the OECD's *Measuring Health Care 1960-1983*[1], in which a substantial effort was made to assure comparability of data through, for example, the use of standard national accounts definitions of spending aggregates, there are still problems of comparability. While these problems have been discussed in detail elsewhere[1,2], it is nevertheless important to keep them in mind when interpreting the results below.

There are also significant conceptual difficulties in making international comparisons of health systems. Even countries at similar stages of economic development differ with respect to various economic and demographic factors, which create problems both of measurement and interpretation. Such factors include differences in: age structures, population density and distribution, cultural attitudes about health and family care, birth and death rates, incidences of morbidity, climate and other environmental factors, industrial and occupational mixes, public and private health insurance coverage, cost-sharing, reimbursement systems, absolute and relative price structures, provision of health-related social services, medical practice patterns and the availability of certain medical technologies, efficiency and productivity, administrative costs, and legal systems. While it is difficult both conceptually and empirically to isolate the individual and often interactive effects of these factors (even within an individual country), their effects individually and collectively do much to determine the levels, composition, concentration, and rate of growth of health expenditures.

In order to provide some insights into cross-country differences in several of these important determinants of health expenditures, cross-national differences in age structures, medical practice patterns, price levels, and concentrations of expenditures are now analysed.

Population Composition

Table 2 displays the population composition of the OECD countries in 1980. Population composition is an important determinant both of health expenditures and the ability of the productive population to support the dependent population. As shown in detail in Chapter 8, medical care expenditures on those 65 and over are on average 4 times greater than expenditures on those under 65. Expenditures on those 75 and older can be more than 7 times greater than on those under 65.

On average 12.2 per cent of the population of the OECD was 65 or over in 1980, ranging from a low of 4.6 per cent in Turkey to 16.2 per cent in Sweden. Similarly for those 75 and over, the OECD average was 4.5, ranging from a low of 1.3 per cent in Turkey to 6.2 in Sweden. The average total dependency ratio (i.e. the ratio of those under 15 years of age and over 64 to those 15-64) was 55.3 per cent, ranging from 47.3 in Finland to 76.3 in Turkey, a country with a very high birth rate. The aged dependency ratio (i.e. the proportion of those 65 and over to those 15-64) varies from 8.2 per cent in Turkey to 25.2 in Sweden, with an OECD average of 18.8. There are clearly major differences in population composition across OECD countries, and hence it could be expected that these would lead to differences in spending patterns. These are considered below.

Table 2

POPULATION COMPOSITION, 1980

	Total Population (000's)	Percent 65	Percent 65	Percent 75	Percent 80	Total Dependency Ratio(a)	Aged Dependency Ratio(b)
Australia	14 719.0	90.7	9.3	3.2	1.5	53.6	14.3
Austria	7 505.0	84.5	15.5	6.0	2.7	56.0	24.1
Belgium	9 859.0	85.7	14.3	5.5	2.5	52.4	21.8
Canada	24 098.5	91.1	8.9	3.1	1.5	47.4	13.1
Denmark	5 124.0	85.8	14.2	5.5	2.6	54.2	22.0
Finland	4 786.9	88.0	12.0	4.1	1.8	47.3	17.7
France	53 788.0	86.3	13.7	5.6	2.7	56.2	21.4
Germany	61 658.0	85.0	15.0	5.5	2.4	50.8	22.7
Greece	9 646.0	86.7	13.3	4.8	2.2	56.6	20.8
Iceland	230.0	90.4	9.6	3.9	2.2	57.5	15.1
Ireland	3 401.0	88.9	11.1	4.1	1.9	72.7	19.1
Italy	56 160.0	86.5	13.5	4.8	2.2	54.5	20.9
Japan	116 701.0	91.0	9.0	3.1	1.4	48.4	13.4
Luxembourg	365.0	86.0	14.0	4.9	2.2	50.8	21.1
Netherlands	14 220.0	88.5	11.5	4.4	2.1	50.6	17.3
New Zealand	3 168.7	90.7	9.3	3.2	1.4	57.3	14.6
Norway	4 093.2	85.4	14.6	5.7	2.7	58.3	23.1
Portugal	9 738.0	89.6	10.4	3.4	1.4	57.4	16.4
Spain	37 458.0	89.1	10.9	3.9	1.7	58.3	17.2
Sweden	8 276.0	83.8	16.2	6.2	2.9	55.6	25.2
Switzerland	6 373.0	85.2	14.8	6.0	2.9	48.9	22.0
Turkey	44 467.9	95.4	4.6	1.3	0.4	76.3	8.2
United Kingdom	55 669.0	85.2	14.8	5.6	2.6	56.1	23.1
United States	227 660.0	88.7	11.3	4.4	2.3	51.1	17.1
OECD Total	779 165.0						
Average		87.8	12.2	4.5	2.1	55.3	18.8

Notes: a) Ratio of those aged 0 - 14 and 65 and over to those aged 15 - 64.
b) Ratio of those aged 65 and over to those aged 15 - 64.

Source: World Population Prospects Estimates and Projections as Assessed in 1982, United Nations, New York, 1985. Medium Variant.

Medical Practice Patterns

Differences in medical practice can also account for differences in medical expenditures among countries. Studies of individual countries as well as comparisons across countries indicate substantial variability in surgery rates as well as differences in average levels both within and among countries. Most of these studies compare surgical rates for well-defined procedures, and attempt to statistically analyse the effects of various economic, demographic and health delivery and financing factors on differences in surgical rates[3].

McPherson et al.[4] have identified eleven factors that could a priori account for differences in surgery rates across geographic areas. These include: age and sex composition; age-specific disease incidence; random variations in morbidity with time and place; availability factors including manpower, hospital bed provision, funding, waiting lists, and methods of payment; clinical judgement; variations in patient demand and expectations; rates of organ removal in previous years; prevailing custom; systematic omissions of operations – private surgery, day care; differences in coding procedures; and inaccuracies in information sources.

Chart 1, reproduced from Notzon et al.[5] provides detailed information on Cesarean (C) section rates for 18 industrialised countries. C-section rates per 100 hospital deliveries varied from 5 in Czechoslovakia and 7 in Austria to 16 in Canada and 18 in the United States, a range between top and bottom of more than 2 to 1. The authors found that differences in Cesarean section rates reflected differences in obstetrical practice, that despite such differences, rates had consistently increased over the past decade in all countries studied, that the rates of increase for most countries had been converging, and that such increases underscored the need for the medical community to consider their appropriateness.

Charts 2 and 2a indicate even greater variability in surgical rates for certain other surgical procedures among the United Kingdom (England and Wales), the United States and Canada. For example, cholecystectomy rates for women in Canada were 5 times the rate in the United Kingdom, while the rate in the United States was 3 times the United Kingdom rate. Hysterectomy rates in the United States were 3 times the rate in the United Kingdom, but only slightly higher than Canada. For certain other procedures such as appendectomy for men and women, there was very little cross-national

Chart 1

CESAREAN SECTION RATES PER 100 HOSPITAL DELIVERIES: SELECTED COUNTRIES, 1981

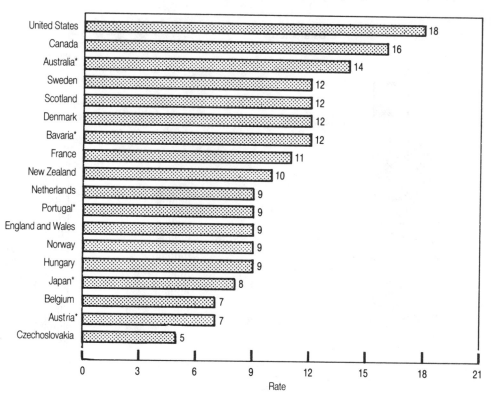

* Incomplete coverage.

Source : Francis C. Notzon, Paul J. Placek, and Selma M. Taffel, "Comparisons of National Cesarean-Section Rates", *The New England Journal of Medicine,* Vol. 316, No. 7, February 12, 1987, p. 387.

variation. Similar results were found in another study comparing New England, England and Norway[6].

There are also significant variations within countries for certain surgical procedures. Chart 3 displays the rates of surgery per 1 000 persons in 44 counties of Ontario, Canada. Variations between highest and lowest rates were generally on the order of 2 to 4-fold, but in several instances exceeded 4-fold. Similarly, a recent study of the United States' Medicare programme of 13 large areas found at least threefold differences in use rates for 67 of the 123 medical and surgical procedures analysed[7].

In general statistical analyses have focused both on differences in the variances of surgical rates and on differences in the average rates *per se*. The results indicate that there is generally consistency across countries in the rank ordering of the procedures displaying the most variation, although the average surgical levels for certain procedures differed across countries. For example, McPherson and Wennberg[8] found that tonsillectomy, hemorrhoidectomy, hysterectomy and

prostatectomy varied more from area to area than did appendectomy, hernia repair or cholecystectomy. Such ordering appears to be related to uncertainty concerning diagnosis and treatment ("Professional Uncertainty Hypothesis") and is not related to delivery systems differences, patient characteristics, access to care or random variations in morbidity. Supply factors (e.g. numbers of surgeons per capita) do, however, appear to be related to differences in average surgery rates, with a stronger relationship found for decentralised entrepreneurial systems such as that in the United States than in centralised, less market-oriented, systems such as that in the United Kingdom. Nevertheless, as Smits[9] points out, variations in medical practice may be acceptable or highly desirable when:

i) they result from uncertainties in medical science regarding appropriate treatment;
ii) a diagnostic or therapeutic modality is in a phase of active dissemination; or
iii) where the variation reflects underlying differences in patients' health status.

17

Chart 2

RATES PER 100 000 POPULATION OF THREE PROCEDURES: ENGLAND/WALES, CANADA AND THE UNITED STATES, 1975

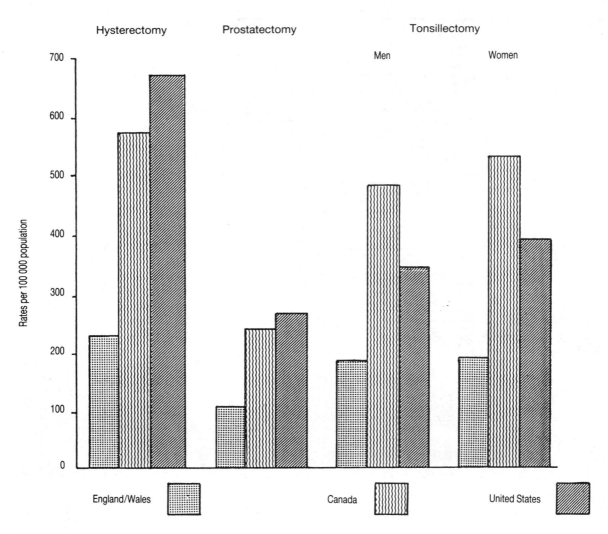

England and Wales, Canada and the United States differ considerably in per-population rates for some common surgical operations. In the mid-1970s, for instance, the differential between England/Wales (E/W) and the United States (US) is nearly 3-fold for hysterectomy and nearly 2.5-fold for prostatectomy.

Source : K. McPherson *et al.,* "Regional Variations in the Use of Common Surgical Procedures: Within and Between England and Wales, Canada and the United States of America", *Social Science and Medicine,* Vol. 15A, 1981, pp. 273-288, in K. Lohr, W. Lohr and R. Brook, *Geographic Variations in the Use of Medical Services and Surgical Procedures: A Chartbook,* National Health Policy Forum, Washington D.C., 1985.

Overall there do appear to be large differences in medical practice patterns both within and across countries which cannot be fully explained on the basis of demographic, economic, or health systems delivery and financing characteristics[10]. However, more troublesome from conceptual and policy perspectives is the great difficulty in measuring the appropriateness of medical care. Without appropriateness criteria, differences in medical practice patterns cannot be assessed in terms of underservice or overservice, *ceteris paribus.*

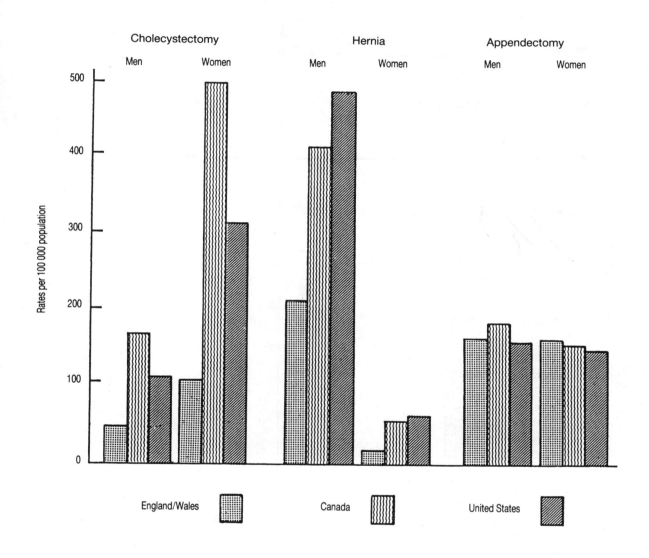

Chart 2 a

RATES PER 100 000 POPULATION OF THREE PROCEDURES: ENGLAND/WALES, CANADA AND THE UNITED STATES, 1975

Among women, cholecystectomy rates varied nearly five-fold between England/Wales and Canada. Other procedures such as appendectomy, however, demonstrated very little cross-national variation.

Source : Same as Chart 2.

Price Levels

International comparisons of health expenditures (indeed of all financial aggregates) are also rendered difficult because overall price levels and relative prices for specific commodities generally differ across countries. The usual procedure in comparing absolute differences in per capita spending across countries is simply to calculate per capita spending in each country, with those figures then converted into a common currency by using

19

Chart 3

RATES PER 1 000 PERSONS OF SEVERAL SURGICAL PROCEDURES
IN 44 COUNTIES OF ONTARIO, CANADA, 1977

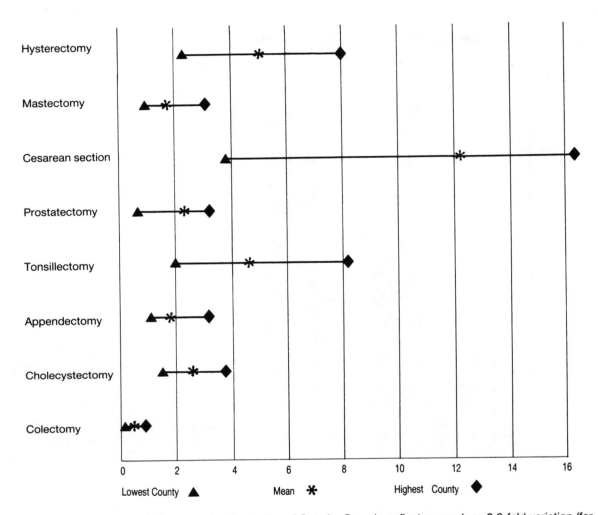

Rates of surgery per 1 000 persons in 44 counties of Ontario, Canada, reflect as much as 9.6-fold variation (for colectomy) and, on the whole, differences of 2- to 4-fold. Such county-level variation is seen for procedures confined to women (hysterectomy, mastectomy, C-sections), those for men (prostatectomy), and those mainly for children (tonsillectomy).

Source : E. Vayda *et al.*, "Five-Year Study of Surgical Rates in Ontario's Counties", *Canadian Medical Association Journal*, Vol. 131, 1985 pp. 111-115, in K. Lohr, W. Lohr and R. Brook, *Geographic Variations in the Use of Medical Services and Surgical Procedures: A Chartbook*, National Health Policy Forum, Washington D.C., 1985.

market exchange rates. However, because market exchange rates do not fully reflect either relative or absolute price differences within countries, the resulting per capita spending figures, when measured in terms of a common currency, reflect not only volume differences but also price differences. In other words, although the exchange-rate-converted expenditures are expressed in

the same currency unit, they are not expressed in the same set of prices. Both the European Community and OECD are currently working on updating the development of price indices, called purchasing power parities (PPPs), which seek to correct for these price differences in exchange-rate-based comparisons.

PPPs are essentially international price indices which

compare the prices of the same set of commodities among different countries. They are in effect exchange rates which express the rate at which one currency should be converted into another in order for a given money expenditure to purchase the same set of goods in both countries[11]. PPPs have been developed for GDP and its components. For health they are the ratio of national average health prices in one country to the corresponding average international prices for the entire comparative group of countries. Dividing expenditures by PPPs results in a measure of volume which reflects the valuation of each countries' health services relative to the average international prices of those services.

Table 3 below contains real per capita health expenditures for 1980 in US$ at: i) average international exchange rates for 1980, ii) using GDP PPPs, and iii) using health PPPs. It also gives the rank ordering of expenditures for 18 OECD countries.

Table 3

PER CAPITA HEALTH EXPENDITURES, 1980

| | On the basis of: | | | | | |
| | Exchange Rates | | GDP PPPs | | Health PPPs | |
Country	$	Rank	$	Rank	$	Rank
United States	1 087	1	1 087	1	809	8
Germany	1 065	2	818	4	825	7
France	1 036	3	837	3	941	2
Netherlands	983	4	773	5	865	3
Norway	963	5	772	6	1 071	1
Denmark	879	6	667	8	665	11
Luxembourg	845	7	714	7	806	9
Canada	787	8	853	2	663	12
Belgium	747	9	596	10	675	10
Austria	718	10	603	9	828	6
Finland	677	11	559	11	853	4
Japan	569	12	537	13	832	5
United Kingdom	530	13	468	15	653	13
Ireland	480	14	510	14	509	15
Italy	479	15	541	12	636	14
Spain	334	16	376	16	405	16
Greece	175	17	211	18	289	18
Portugal	151	18	238	17	375	17

Note: PPPs are purchasing power parities. See text for explanation.

Sources: Measuring Health Care 1960-1983, OECD, Paris, 1985.
National Accounts, Main Aggregates, Volume I, OECD, Paris, 1986.
Michael Ward, Purchasing Power Parities and Real Expenditures in the OECD, OECD, Paris, 1985.

There are significant differences in both absolute amounts of spending and the rank ordering of countries. On the basis of exchange rates the United States, Germany and France had the highest per capita health spending, while Spain, Greece and Portugal had the lowest. When GDP PPPs are used the three highest countries are the United States, Canada and France, while Spain, Greece and Portugal remain the lowest. On the basis of health PPPs Norway, France and the Netherlands are the highest, and Spain, Portugal and Greece again are the lowest. There are also some other significant changes in the distribution, such as Japan moving from 12th (exchange rates) and 13th (GDP PPPs) to fifth. Moreover, the absolute differences among the highest and lowest expenditure countries are narrowed, because countries with higher overall and/or

higher health prices tend to be the higher expenditure countries, and conversely.

Concentration of Spending

Another important aspect of individual country's health systems that has important implications for international comparisons of delivery systems, financing, and overall expenditures is the concentration of expenditures on relatively small numbers of individuals: the aged, persons in their last year(s) of life, and individuals with heavy prior use of services. While detailed data are not available for many countries on the concentration of spending, the available data and casual evidence suggest that there are some important similarities among countries. For example, per capita expenditures for the aged are on average four times those for the non-aged.

Data on cumulative spending distributions (e.g. cumulative proportions of those eligible/protected compared with cumulative percentages of spending) also indicate similar patterns of concentration across countries. Tables 4 and 5 contain cumulative spending information for the United States' Medicare programme and for France's Caisse Nationale de l'Assurance Maladie[12]. The populations are clearly not demographically equivalent, because the Medicare data are only for aged enrollees, whereas the Caisse Nationale covers all age groups. Both studies contain information on cumulative spending for programme eligibles, and compare changes in spending concentrations over time.

The United States data indicate that in 1982 2 per cent of eligibles accounted for 31.9 per cent of total spending, 5 per cent of eligibles accounted for 54 per cent, and 8.8 per cent of eligibles accounted for 70.6 per cent of total spending. The top 2 per cent of eligibles had average reimbursements of $23 818, and the top 4 per cent utilisation group of eligibles had reimbursements of $17 897, compared with $1 469 for all aged enrollees. At the other end of the distribution 38.9 per cent of eligibles used no services, and 89 per cent of eligibles accounted

Table 4

CONCENTRATION OF UNITED STATES MEDICARE EXPENDITURES, 1982
(Cumulative Percentages)

Eligibles	Expenditures
0.5	12.5
1.0	20.3
2.0	31.9
2.8	39.1
4.0	47.9
5.0	54.0
5.8	58.4
8.8	70.6
11.0	77.1
61.1	100
100.0	100

Source: Gerald Riley, James Lubitz, Ronald Prihoda, and Mary Ann Stevenson, "Changes in Distribution of Medicare Expenditures Among Aged Enrollees, 1969-82", Health Care Financing Review, Spring 1986, p. 55.

for only 22.9 per cent of spending. The study also found that the concentration of spending in 1982 was similar to the distributions in 1969 and 1975, although there had been a slight decrease in the concentration of spending over this period.

The information from France provides a similar picture. The highest 5 per cent of eligibles accounted for 63.5 per cent of expenditures, compared with 54 per cent in the United States. This greater concentration in the French distribution may be due to differences in the population, in particular the inclusion of the non-aged and hence expenditures on traumatic accidents and intensive birth-related services for the young. On the other hand, 23 per cent of persons consumed no services in 1980, the lowest 40 per cent of eligibles accounted for just 0.4 per cent of expenditures, 55 per cent accounted for 2.5 per cent of expenditures, and 75 per cent accounted for 10.8 per cent of spending.

Two other interesting aspects of the French studies are the sensitivity of the spending distribution to the time period chosen, and changes in the distribution over time. The time period is evidently important in two ways. First, over a longer time period (e.g. three years as compared with one year), a greater proportion (95 versus 77 per cent) of the population consumes services, because the probability of needing some medical care increases with the time span. Second, there is greater concentration in the distribution of spending over a shorter period. For example, data from the study by the *Caisse Nationale de l'Assurance Maladie* show that over a one-year period (1980) 2.5 per cent of the population accounted for half of all spending. However, if a three-year time period is taken (1978-80), 4 per cent of eligibles accounted for 50 per cent of spending. This occurs because shorter time periods result in greater concentration in the distribution as a result of greater weight given to costly but time-limited acute care (e.g. traumatic accidents). In particular, specific acute care cases which require costly short-term hospitalisation with little or no follow-up care tend to have a more significant weight over a one-year period, because amortising these costs over three years reduces their weight in the upper end of the distribution.

In analysing changes in the distribution between two points in time, a comparison of spending concentrations in 1970 and 1980 showed, contrary to the United States

Table 5

CONCENTRATION OF FRENCH MEDICAL EXPENDITURES, 1980-81
(Cumulative Percentages)

Eligibles	Expenditures
0.1	5.7
5.0	63.5
10.0	73.7
15.0	80.5
20.0	85.4
25.0	89.2
30.0	92.2
35.0	94.4
40.0	96.2
45.0	97.5
50.0	98.6
55.0	99.3
60.0	99.6
77.0	100
100	100

Sources: An. Mizrahi and Ar. Mizrahi, Débours et Dépenses Médicales Selon l'Age et le Sexe -- France -- 1970-1980, Centre de Recherche, d'Etude et de Documentation en Economie de la Santé, Paris, 1985, p. 23; and Qui Consomme Quoi?, Caisse Nationale de l'Assurance Maladie des Travailleurs Salariés, Paris, 1982, p. 10.

study, a small increase in concentration over this ten-year period. Nevertheless, in neither study does there appear to have been a significant increase in the relative resource use (e.g. concentration of spending) for the most critically ill. Such a result is counter to the conventional wisdom that use of new costly life-saving and life-sustaining technologies for the most critically ill has been one of the most important factors in the recent growth of health care expenditure.

Other studies have also shown high costs associated with the last years of life. For example, 6 per cent of United States Medicare beneficiaries in their last year of life accounted for almost 30 per cent of total spending. Studies in a number of countries have also found a strong relationship between prior and current use of health services[13].

These concentrations of spending result from both the unequal distribution of needs across population groups as well as the financing and delivery systems within individual countries. While in all countries certain groups will have higher medical care needs than does the "average" citizen, differences in these relative spending patterns, as well as concentrations of spending distributions across countries, will also depend on specific features of the financing and delivery systems.

NOTES AND REFERENCES

1. *Measuring Health Care 1960-1983*, OECD, Paris, 1985.

2. Robert A. Maxwell, *Health and Wealth: An International Study of Health Care Spending*, Lexington Books, Lexington, Massachusetts, 1981; and Brian Abel-Smith (ed.), *Eurocare*, Health Econ, Basle, Switzerland.

3. For two of the most comprehensive studies, see Henry J. Aaron and William B. Schwartz, *The Painful Prescription Rationing Hospital Care*, The Brookings Institution, Washington D.C., 1984; and J.W. Hurst, *Financing Health Services in the United States, Canada, and Britain*, King Edward's Hospital Fund, London, 1985.

4. Klim McPherson *et al.*, "Regional Variations in the Use of Common Surgical Procedures: Within and Between England and Wales, Canada, and the United States of America", *Social Science and Medicine*, Vol. 15A, 1981, p. 274.

5. Francis C. Notzon, Paul J. Placek and Selma M. Taffel, "Comparisons of National Cesarean-Section Rates", *The New England Journal of Medicine*, Vol. 316, No. 7, Feb. 12, 1987.

6. Klim McPherson *et al.*, "Small-Area Variations in the Use of Common Surgical Procedures: An International Comparison of New England, England, and Norway", *The New England Journal of Medicine*, Vol. 307, No. 21, Nov. 18, 1982; and John E. Wennberg and Marian Gornick, *A Study of the Nature, Causes and Cost Implications of Hospital Market Variations in Use of Inpatient Services*, Staff Summary No. 84-1, United States Department of Health and Human Services, Health Care Financing Administration, Baltimore, Maryland, 1984.

7. Mark R. Chassin *et al.*, "Variations in the Use of Medical and Surgical Services by the Medicare Population", *The New England Journal of Medicine*, Vol. 314, No. 5, Jan. 30, 1986.

8. Klim McPherson *et al.*, "Small-Area Variations in the Use of Common Surgical Procedures: An International Comparison of New England, England, and Norway", *op.cit.*; Kathleen N. Lohr, William R. Lohr, and Robert H. Brook, *Geographic Variations in the Use of Medical Services and Surgical Procedures A Chartbook*, National Health Policy Forum, Washington, D.C., October 1985; and John E. Wennberg and Marian Gornick, *A Study of the Nature, Causes and Cost Implications of Hospital Market Variations in Use of Inpatient Services*, *op.cit.*

9. Helen L. Smits, "Medical Practice Variations Revisited", *Health Affairs*, Fall 1986.

10. For a review of the relevant literature, see *CCC Bibliography on Regional Variations in Health Care 1985*, Copenhagen Collaborating Centre, Copenhagen, 1985; *Health Affairs*, Summer 1984; and Tavs Andersen, "Variations in Common Medical Practice: Some Economic Challenges", Internal Working Paper, OECD, Paris, 1987.

11. See Michael Ward, *Purchasing Power Parities and Real Expenditures in the OECD*, OECD, Paris, 1985.

12. See Gerald Riley *et al.*, "Changes in Distribution of Medicare Expenditures Among Aged Enrollees, 1969-82", *Health Care Financing Review*, Spring 1986; *Qui Consomme Quoi?*, Caisse Nationale de l'Assurance Maladie des Travailleurs Salariés, Paris, 1982; and An. Mizrahi and Ar. Mizrahi, *Débours et Dépenses Médicales Selon l'Age et le Sexe*, Centre de Recherche, d'Etude et de Documentation en Economie de la Santé, Paris, 1985.

13. See A. Dale Tussing, *Irish Medical Care Resources: An Economic Analysis*, The Economic and Social Research Institute, Dublin, Ireland, 1985; J. Lubitz and R. Prihoda, "The Use and Costs of Medicare Services in the Last 2 Years of Life", *Health Care Financing Review*, Spring 1984; and Nobuo Maeda, "Medical Care Costs for the Aged in Japan", Paper presented at the XIIIe International Congress of Gerontology, July 1985, New York.

Chapter 3

THE HEALTH SYSTEMS OF OECD COUNTRIES

This chapter describes the institutional features of the health care financing and delivery systems in the OECD. The health care systems of OECD countries appear to be structurally diverse and based on different underlying philosophical principles[1]. Nevertheless, despite these differences, there are important similarities among the systems, and most of the systems face similar financing and delivery problems due to structural inefficiencies and often perverse economic incentives.

The health care systems of OECD countries can be characterised in a variety of ways, none of which is mutually exhaustive or wholly analytically satisfying. One possible dichotomy is to classify systems in terms of consumer sovereignty as compared with social equity models, the former being characterised by incentives, the latter by control. The most frequent approach categorises systems according to one of three basic models:

  i)   the National Health Service [Beveridge] model, characterised by universal coverage, national general tax financing, and national ownership and/or control of the factors of production;

  ii) the Social Insurance [Bismarck] model, characterised by compulsory universal coverage generally within the framework of Social Security, and financed by employer and individual contributions through non-profit insurance funds, and public and/or private ownership of factors of production; and

  iii) the private insurance (consumer sovereignty) model, characterised by employer-based or individual purchase of private health insurance coverage financed by individual and/or employer contributions and private ownership of the factors of production[2].

The prototypical country examples of these systems are: National Health Service model – the United Kingdom, Italy; Social Insurance model – France, Germany; Private Insurance model – the United States.

In fact, because of the large diversities both among and within OECD health systems, none of these models provides a wholly adequate description. For example, private insurance and private ownership of the factors of production are found in the United Kingdom; major public programmes and public ownership exist in the United States; Japan has a compulsory national system that relies heavily on employer-based coverage. Switzerland does not have a federal health insurance system (except for accident insurance), although some cantons require coverage of certain population subgroups (e.g. children) and overall 98 per cent of the population voluntarily purchase insurance which is often publicly underwritten. Similarly, in the Netherlands a combination of public health insurance programmes covers some 70 per cent of the population (i.e. employees and the elderly with incomes below certain levels and other low income individuals), while those not covered by public insurance may take out private insurance. In addition, all individuals, regardless of income, are insured against catastrophic medical expenses.

Perhaps of more importance is the similarity of objectives and the economic incentives inherent in these diverse systems. The basic objective of all these systems is the provision of access to quality care for all citizens while achieving efficiency in the use and provision of services. All systems attempt to achieve allocational efficiency and distributional equity. They also contain implicit or explicit employment and sometimes balance of payments incentives.

It is of course difficult to measure achievement of distributional and allocational goals. Defining distributional equity involves normative judgement, and definition and measurement of "equality of access" is problematic[3]. Measurement of allocational efficiency requires the measurement of health outcomes and the relating of expenditures on health to improvements in outcomes. As discussed in the next chapter, both are difficult to achieve.

In attempting on *a priori* grounds to evaluate the performance of different health systems, it is useful to analyse the implicit and explicit incentives inherent in their structural and financing characteristics. Generically these would include financing procedures, eligibility criteria, benefits provided, reimbursement procedures and organisation and development of the delivery system.

Financing

Financing procedures affect the redistributive impact of the system, the allocation of resources, and overall economic growth. Public and private health care financing systems are designed to spread the financial consequences associated with ill-health over large population groups. The group can be the population of a geographic entity such as an entire country, an employment-related group, an individual insurance fund's membership, groups of individuals with similar characteristics, etc. In most OECD countries, the individual's ability to pay relative to needs is taken into account implicitly (progressivity of tax systems) or explicitly (waivers of cost-sharing, income-related contributions, spreading additional health care costs of pensioners across the entire population) in the establishment of individual contribution levels[4].

Health care systems can be financed through general taxes (personal income, corporate profit, VAT, sales), specific taxes (e.g. excise taxes on specific commodities, taxes of specific factors of production), premiums, user charges (co-insurance and deductibles), and charitable contributions[5]. The specific combination of methods used will determine the distributional impact of the financing of the health system (including intergenerational redistribution), the sensitivity of the financing base to changes in the overall economy ("revenue elasticity" of the financing base), and could affect both the supply and demand for labour and capital and their use in production. Most countries in fact use combinations of these methods, with countries such as the United Kingdom and Italy relying heavily on general taxes, France, Belgium and Luxembourg on payroll taxes, and the United States, Japan and Switzerland on employer and/or employee premiums. Unfortunately the information does not at present exist to attribute these financing costs across income classes for the OECD countries[6].

Eligibility

Eligibility criteria differ among countries. However, given the near universal coverage under public and/or private systems in OECD countries, the few differences among countries are not great. Most systems cover employees, their families, pensioners, and disadvantaged groups. There are differences in eligibility for certain groups such as students, those never in the labour force, the long-term unemployed, individuals who can (or must) opt out of the system, etc. However, those not covered under public or private systems can generally receive care in publicly-operated health care facilities or through religious or other charitable institutions.

Public coverage data presented in Chapter 5 indicate that in 1983 in 20 of the 23 OECD countries (excluding Turkey) for which data are available, at least 95 per cent of the population is eligible for public coverage against the risk of hospitalisation. Spain is phasing in a national health service that will ultimately cover the entire population, and in the Netherlands and the United States the great majority of those without public coverage have private insurance. Unfortunately, there is little readily-accessible cross-country data on the penetration and extensiveness of benefits of private health insurance coverage[7]. Further, coverage by public programmes does not necessarily imply appropriate use of services. Even in countries with universal coverage there are still concerns about the utilisation rates of certain socio-economic groups, despite significant improvements in access over the past twenty years[8].

Benefits

The particular benefits covered under public and private health systems also differ. Hospital inpatient services, inpatient physician services, and outpatient physician and diagnostic services are covered under virtually all programmes. For drugs, eyeglasses, hearing aids, nursing homes, home health, and health-related social services there is far more diversity. In some countries, such as Belgium and Ireland, specific benefits covered depend on the income level or employment status of the individual. In certain countries, such as Germany and Finland, social service provision is a regional or local as opposed to a national responsibility. In addition, due to differences in both implicit and explicit policy choices as well as differences in medical practice, there are numerous differences across countries in the conditions under which certain services are covered (e.g. age restrictions for chronic renal dialysis, exclusion of chronic alcoholics from liver transplants). If cost-sharing is regarded as a benefit reduction (as opposed to a financing mechanism), fundamental differences can also be seen in benefits as a result of differences in cost-sharing among countries. In France, Belgium, Japan and the United States cost-sharing applies to most services under public programmes. In the United Kingdom, the Scandinavian countries, the Netherlands, Spain, Switzerland, Canada and Germany significant cost-sharing on basic services is generally perceived as inconsistent with the underlying social welfare aims of the public health programmes. However, virtually all countries impose cost-sharing on pharmaceuticals. Interestingly, virtually all countries waive cost-sharing for the poor, and some impose limits on cumulative cost-sharing payments. Moreover, as discussed in Chapter 9, cost-sharing levels are generally quite nominal.

All countries also provide individual and collective benefits through their public health systems. All undertake basic public health measures concerning environment, transmission of contagious diseases, approval of pharmaceuticals, medical research and education, immunisation programmes, pre- and post-natal care, anti-smoking, drug, and alcohol abuse programmes, etc. There are, however, differences in resource commitments and emphases. For example, Japan emphasizes fitness programmes, and has special public programmes for those suffering from nuclear irradiation. While precise comparative information on these programmes is not readily available, expenditures on those activities are included in the spending aggregates analysed below. Furthermore, it must be remembered that these public health (as opposed to strictly social insurance) efforts have significant impacts on mortality, morbidity, and life expectancy, and hence on overall economic performance and social expenditures.

Reimbursement

The methods by which medical care providers are paid for services rendered have major influences on access, cost and quality of care. Even in systems with closed-ended financing, payment methods influence the allocation of resources within the overall limits, and hence can result in differing quantities and qualities of service being provided for the same level of expenditure. Furthermore, the actual flows of funds themselves contain inherent incentives for both the demand and supply of services. Thus, the incentives inherent in direct reimbursement systems such as those in Germany and Japan, where the reimbursement flows from the insurance funds to medical care providers, may be very different from the indemnity approaches in Belgium and France, where the patient pays the medical care provider and is reimbursed by the insurance fund. Furthermore, it is important to focus on the interactions among reimbursement mechanisms. For example, the payment mechanism for hospitals may well have intended or unintended effects on both the supply and demand for physician services.

The scope of control over the system is also of critical importance. Systems in which reimbursement methods and levels are coordinated allow incentives to affect the entire system. Fragmented systems characterised by unequal power among reimbursing entities and providers are less likely to achieve overall objectives of systems efficiency. In fact, this is the very problem facing private health insurers in Europe. Given the relatively small sizes of the funds, the large numbers of providers, the competitive marketing of policies which necessitates that insurees have broad freedom of choice of provider, and the extremely limited share of private insurance in total health spending, effective cost containment in the private sector is difficult.

Reimbursement systems among OECD countries differ widely. In attempting both to control expenditure increases and to obtain more efficient resource use out of existing expenditure levels, many countries have recently modified their reimbursement procedures[9]. Because, as discussed below, much of the increase in

spending is due to increased utilisation and intensity of services, considerable emphasis has been placed on systems that limit quantity and total expenditure as well as prices.

Because hospital expenditures are the largest expenditure item, there has been much emphasis on hospital payment. Public systems and private insurers use a variety of methods to pay hospitals. Most are prospective in nature[10]. These approaches can be summarised along the three dimensions of the base of compensation (e.g. unit of payment), process for determining the payment level, and whether the established levels apply to individual or groups of hospitals[11]. Regarding the rate basis for hospitals, four different bases are generally used: annual budgets (global or line-by-line), and payments per day, per case (e.g. Diagnosis Related Groups – DRGs), and per unit of service. Reimbursement levels can be established under a variety of mechanisms including: being unilaterally established by public authority, insurance carrier, or provider; negotiated among various relevant parties; and determined by market forces (including competitive bidding). Furthermore the resulting payments can be hospital-specific or apply to groups of (or indeed all) hospitals. Different methods may be used by different payers (e.g. public vs. private), and various components of hospitals (e.g. inpatient care, outpatient care, operating costs, capital costs, medical education, physician services, etc.) may be reimbursed differently.

Table 6 summarises the hospital reimbursement systems in several OECD countries. In a number of them, the United Kingdom, Germany and France (public hospitals), the payment to the hospital also generally includes reimbursement for all physician services. In other countries, such as the United States, most Canadian provinces, Japan, and France (private hospitals) separate fee-for-service payments are generally made to physicians. Separation of physician and hospital payment often depends on whether the hospital is a public or private one (e.g. France, United Kingdom). Private insurance in most countries reimburses hospitals and physicians separately. While it is not easy to generalise about incentive effects given this plethora of systems, the following types of effects are generally consistent with *a priori* expectations and observed behaviour. Annual budgets have the advantage of simplicity and overall expenditure control, but do not necessarily provide strong incentives for micro-efficiency or quality. *Per diem* payments also have the advantage of simplicity and fewer disincentives than global budgets from quantity and quality perspectives, but since *per diem* payment systems provide incentives for increased length of stay per admission, they do not (in the absence of volume controls) provide incentives for limiting overall expenditures. Per case (or diagnosis) payments have incentives for reduced length of stay per case, but also provide incentives for increased admissions and possible reductions in quality or service intensity per case. If the payments do not adequately reflect resource use (and implicitly case severity), such systems may also provide disincentives to treat complex cases. Fee-for-service provides strong incentives for service provision and quality and through adjustments of relative fees can promote allocational goals at a very micro level, but contains disincentives from an overall expenditure perspective unless accompanied by strong volume controls. Thus, it would be expected, *a priori*, that prospective total budget approaches inclusive of inpatient physician services such as the British National Health Service would result in lower expenditures than would a retrospective *per diem* cost or charge-based system with physicians being paid on a fee-for-service basis. In fact, most OECD countries have implemented, or are moving towards, either total budget approaches (the United Kingdom, Canada, France) or prospective *per diem* (Germany) or per case (the United States) systems.

Physician expenditures are generally the second largest health expenditure category, and in their role as the central decision-maker in virtually all health systems, physicians' decisions affect the great majority of health expenditures. Thus, the incentives inherent in physician payment systems are critical in determining overall systems costs.

There is considerable diversity of physician payment systems both among and within most OECD countries. Several different methods are used within most countries to pay physicians. Sometimes these methods depend on the place of service, payer category, specialty of the physician, geographic location, type of insurance contract, physician participation status, etc. The general payment methods employed are capitation, salary, and variants of fee-for-service (e.g. fee schedules; usual, customary, and reasonable charges; actual charges), as well as combinations of these methods (e.g. capitation and fee-for-service for Danish primary care physicians outside Copenhagen). Payments by case (e.g. physician DRGs) are currently under study, although not in general use. Payment levels and relative prices (or remuneration) can be established unilaterally or through negotiations among governmental entities, social insurance funds, private insurers, physicians, consumers and/or employers[12]. Many countries have different payment systems for hospital-based as opposed to ambulatory care physicians. Some systems employ ambulatory care physicians, usually general practitioners, as "gatekeepers" for consumers to access hospitals, tests, social services, etc. Some systems allow patient freedom of choice of physician, while others require individuals to choose a single primary-care physician.

Table 7 summarises the physician payment methods in the seven major OECD countries. In the United States, Belgium, France, Germany, Japan, Ireland and Switzerland ambulatory physician services are generally reimbursed on a fee-for-service basis. In the United Kingdom, Spain, the Netherlands [public system], and

Table 6

HOSPITAL REIMBURSEMENT AND FINANCING IN SELECTED OECD COUNTRIES

Country	Ownership of hospitals	Basis of Reimbursement For: Operating costs	Basis of Reimbursement For: Capital costs	The role of health sector planning
Canada	Predominantly by lay boards of trustees or by communities.	Annual prospective global budgets controlled by the provincial governments.	Separate capital budgets granted, upon specific approval of proposed investments, by the provincial government.	The hospital sector is subject to planning by the provincial government. The capacity of the system is fully determined by the provincial governments.
United Kingdom	Central government's National Health Service.	Annual prospective global budgets controlled by the National Health Service (i.e. the central government).	Separate capital budgets controlled by the central government through the National Health Service.	Regional and District Health Authorities develop health plans. Because the National Health Service owns all but the few private hospitals, the Health Authorities and central government fully determine the capacity of the hospital system.
France	About 70% of all hospital beds are publicly owned (mainly by local governments); the rest are privately owned.	Prior to 1984 prospective per diems and prospectively set charges for particular services. These payments were government controlled. After 1983 prospectively set global budgets.	Capital costs are recovered in part through amortization allowances in the per diems and charges. The balance of costs are financed through subsidies from the central and local governments.	The hospital sector is subject to regional and national planning. The central government, through its health plan, determines the capacity of the hospital system.
Netherlands	Local communities or lay boards of trustees.	Until 1983 by negotiated per diems and charges; since 1984, by annual global budgets.	Until 1983, the per diems included amortization of capital costs. Since 1983, hospitals are reimbursed for capital costs via separately controlled line items in the budget.	Construction of facilities and acquisition of major medical equipment requires a government-issued license, which is issued on the basis of regional and national health-sector planning.
Sweden	Owned and operated by local community councils.	Annual budgets, controlled by the local community councils.	Community-financed, by means of specific appropriations voted by the community councils.	The capacity of the hospital sector is planned and controlled at the community level. There is no formal national health plan.
Finland	Owned and operated by local communities.	Annual budgets, determined by a system of national health planning and ultimately controlled by the central government.	Specific appropriations; financed in part by the communities and in part by central government subsidy.	There is a system of national health planning, ultimately controlled by the central government. A system of central government subsidies effectively controls the capacity of the hospital system.

Table 6 (Cont'd)

Country	Ownership of hospitals	Basis of Reimbursement For:		The role of health sector planning
		Operating costs	Capital costs	
Germany	Owned by local communities, by religious foundations, or by private individuals (usually physicians).	Prospective, hospital speci-fic, all-inclusive per diems negotiated between the hos-pital & regional associations of sickness funds. These rates are subject to approval by the state governments.	Financed by the federal and state governments through lump sum grants (for short-lived equipment) or upon specific application (for structures or long-lived equipment).	Capital investments are approved and financed by the state governments on the basis of state-wide hospital planning. The state governments therefore control the capacity of the hospital system.
Japan	All hospitals are non-profit. Over 60 per cent of all hospital beds are privately owned (most by individuals or groups of physicians). The rest are public.	Fee-for-service	Capital costs are met through the fee-for-service payments. For private hospitals, public loan schemes for initial capital costs are available. For public hospitals, initial capital costs are met through governmental grants.	All facilities must meet general certifi-cation requirements stipulated in the national Medical Supply Law. While all hospitals must have a permit from the Pre-fectural government, only public hospitals can be denied a permit if the additional bed capacity would result in a bed supply in excess of the established targets.
United States	Over 60 per cent of all hospital beds are privately owned; 85 per cent are non-profit. The remainder are owned by federal, state and local governments.	Prior to 1984, the federal Medicare for the aged and disabled reimbursed hospitals on the basis of retrospectively-determined reasonable costs. Since 1984 reimbursement is on the basis of prospectively-established payments per case (Diagnosis Related Groups-DRGs). Individual state Medicaid Programme(s) use a variety of systems. Private insurers use a variety of approaches, predominantly retrospective cost or charge based.	Under Medicare capital is currently reimbursed on a retrospective reasonable cost basis; but in the future is likely to be blended into the DRG rate. For other payors, reimbursement for capital is generally included in the payment rate. The principal governmental subsidies for capital are through the tax exemption of financing instruments for health care institutions.	Planning is undertaken at state and local levels with some federal financial support. In most states and localities hospitals must obtain a "certificate of need" for opening of new beds or major acquisitions of equipment.

Sources: Uwe E. Reinhardt, "Access, Quality and Efficiency: Hospitals and Other Institutional Services", Health and Pension Policies Under Economic and Demographic Constraints, OECD, Paris, 1987.
Information on Japan and the United States provided by the OECD Secretariat.

Denmark (in Copenhagen) patients select a G.P. as their principal physician who is reimbursed on a capitation basis. Both reimbursement procedures and traditional place of treatment for ambulatory care services can have significant effects both on physician and on overall health systems costs. For example, in Sweden about 60 per cent of ambulatory care services are provided in public clinics or hospitals by salaried physicians, whereas in Germany virtually all ambulatory care is provided in physicians' private offices. In Ireland physi-cians providing ambulatory care in hospitals are salar-ied, while those in private offices are paid on a fee-for-service basis. In the United Kingdom, Germany, France (public hospitals) and Ireland (public patients) physician compensation is included in the hospital reimbursement, and physicians are generally salaried. In the United States, France (private hospitals), Bel-gium, Luxembourg, and Japan physician services to hospital patients are generally reimbursed on a fee-for-service base. In the United States, France (non-convention), and Australia physicians can charge patients in excess of the established reimbursement amounts. In several countries private insurance is prohibited from filling in these gaps (or the requisite cost-sharing amounts). Canada recently passed a law reducing federal health grants to provinces on a one-to-one basis for physicians' extra-billing of patients.

The incentives inherent in these systems are some-what different. Simplistically stated, fee-for-service payment provides strong incentives for provision of additional services, high quality and increased expendi-tures. Salary reimbursement contains incentives for reduced service provision, potentially lower quality, and reduced expenditures. Case payments, such as physician DRGs, provide incentives for efficiency by attempting to equate reimbursement to "output", but are difficult (perhaps not feasible) to establish technically, and can result in administrative problems when several physi-cians are involved in treating a particular case. Capita-tion provides incentives to reduce quantities and expen-ditures while maintaining the patients' health status. But salary, case payments and capitation contain strong incentives for referral to other entities or use of certain ancillary or other non-physician services, provided the referring physician's remuneration is not reduced. How-ever, to the extent the capitated entity (e.g. prepaid group) is financially responsible for all care for the patient, overall spending may be reduced. In certain countries such as Canada (in certain provinces) and Germany, either individual physician or geographical expenditure limits have been set to offset the inherent quantity escalation incentives in fee-for-service, while maintaining its inherent allocational incentives.

In summary, on *a priori* grounds, it would be expected

Table 7

PHYSICIAN REIMBURSEMENT SYSTEMS IN THE MAJOR SEVEN OECD COUNTRIES

	Country	Ambulatory Sector	Hospital Sector
General Practitioners	Canada	Fee-for-service Salary (health centres)	Fee-for-service (self-employed physicians) Salary (employed physicians)
	France	Fee-for-service Salary (in health centres)	Salary (public hospitals) Fee-for-service (private hospitals)
	Italy	Capitation plus special allocations	Salary
	Japan	Fee-for-service	Fee-for-service

	United Kingdom	Capitation plus
		  fee-for-service for
		  certain preventive
		  procedures plus
		  special allocations
			Salary
			
			Fee-for-Service
			  (private hospitals)

	United States	Fee-for-service Capitation	Fee-for-service Salary
	Germany	Fee-for-service	Salary (when in training)
Specialists	Canada	Fee-for-service Salary (health centres)	Fee-for-service (self-employed physicians) Salary (employed physicians)
	France	Fee-for-service Salary (in health centres)	Salary (public hospitals) Fee-for-service (private hospitals)
	Italy	Salary (in health centres) Fee-for service (private offices)	Salary
	Japan	Fee-for-service	Fee-for-service

	United Kingdom	Salary plus
		  fee-for-service for
		  home visits
			Salary
			
			Fee-for-service
			  (private hospitals)

	United States	Fee-for-service Capitation, Salary	Fee-for-service Salary

	Germany	Fee-for-service	Salary (the rule)
			
			Fee-for service, for private
			  patients treated by chiefs
			  of departments

Sources: Uwe Reinhardt: The Compensation of Physicians: The Experience Abroad, Report prepared for the U.S. Health Care Financing Administration, Washington D.C., 1985.
The Japanese Ministry of Health and Welfare, "Outline of Recent Japanese Policy on Health: The Background and Measures for Reform", in Health and Pension Policies Under Economic and Demographic Constraints, OECD, Paris, 1987.

that countries with higher public penetration and capitation or salary reimbursement for ambulatory care would have relatively lower ambulatory care expenditures than would open-ended fee-for-service systems. Similarly, it would be expected that institutional physician expenditures would be lower where physicians are salaried or capitated as compared with a fee-for-service system. On the other hand, to the extent that capitation and salary for ambulatory care result in more frequent testing, use of drugs, and/or hospitalisation (if the capitated or salaried entity is not at risk), expenditures for these items may tend to be higher than in a fee-for-service system. Quality of care may also be affected under these arrangements.

Pharmaceuticals are also a significant expenditure item. Reimbursement is generally on a fee-for-service basis. Pharmaceuticals supplied to institutionalised individuals are usually considered as part of the institutional service and are included in the institution's reimbursement. Fees are established on the basis of a number of criteria, including retail price, wholesale prices, acquisition costs, etc. Fees are often based on the prices of the lowest cost generic equivalent. Reimbursement is generally made to the pharmacist directly or to the patient. In a limited number of cases (e.g. Switzerland, Japan) physicians can be reimbursed directly for pharmaceuticals supplied to patients. Increases in, and the level of, pharmaceutical expenditures have posed a significant budgetary problem in several OECD countries. For example inpatient and outpatient pharmaceuticals account for over 30 per cent of Japanese health expenditures. Much of the activity on pharmaceuticals has centred on increasing cost-sharing, substituting lower-cost generic equivalents, and removing certain drugs from coverage. Reimbursement measures have also been designed to reduce payments either at the wholesale or the retail level, and in a limited number of cases to promote competitive bidding and bulk purchasing. The pharmaceutical industry has been partially nationalised in Sweden.

It is difficult to discuss reimbursement practices for nursing homes, home health services, hospices, other health-related social services, and other health services and supplies, because definitions and practices differ substantially across countries, and their is a dearth of reliable comparable information. However, in a number of countries coverage and reimbursement systems strongly favour institution-based long-term care services over home and community-based care. As discussed below, expenditures on these services could be expected to increase as populations age and disease patterns change. While on *a priori* grounds total budget and prospective payment systems for nursing homes and other forms of institutionalised long-term care would appear to contain appropriate efficiency incentives, quality assurance is a more fundamental problem, because many of the medical safeguards (e.g. extensive physician involvement) inherent in acute medical care

largely are missing in the treatment of long-term chronic illness.

Organisation and Development of the Delivery System

The overall organisation and development of health care delivery systems play a fundamental role in determining costs, access and quality. Specific characteristics would include: whether the resource commitment is open- or closed-ended; quality assurance mechanisms; if (and how) ownership, allocation and distribution of health facilities, equipment and manpower are planned centrally, locally, left to the working of the market, and/or based on a combination of all these factors; the legal structure of the country concerning malpractice costs, anti-trust litigation, federal-local legal responsibilities, the spectrum of medical care providers and alternative permissible delivery arrangements, and the legally permissible types of business arrangements. These characteristics of health care systems interact, and have a major impact on financing, quality, reimbursement, eligibility and benefits.

The open- or closed-ended nature of the system fundamentally affects overall costs, reimbursement and quality. Systems which are basically closed-ended, such as the National Health Service in the United Kingdom[13], or systems which establish a fixed limit on federal financing to regions, such as Canada, could be expected more effectively to limit overall health spending than would systems which are based heavily on market principles. However, spending is only one dimension of a health care system, and it is also necessary to evaluate the effects on quality of care and health outcomes and whether costs are being shifted to other governmental units, medical care providers, or consumers of care[14].

Quality assurance is difficult to define and measure. Quality assurance spans a wide range of activities from licensing requirements, educational requirements for professional medical and para-medical personnel, life-safety code standards, peer review, and various other utilisation review mechanisms. Quality standards are enforced through on-site inspections, examination of patients and/or medical records by peer review and governmental organisations, pre-admission, concurrent, and post-discharge review, retrospective claims review and action taken by governmental agencies and medical organisations on an individual or class-action complaint basis.

At a very micro level utilisation review can focus on: comparing medical charts against pre-established indicators of sub-standard care; inpatient reviews of readmissions within 14 days of discharge, surgical related deaths, neurological deficit related to anesthesia, organ failure not present at admission, and post-operative and post-procedure complications; appropriateness and quality of surgical services through reviews of samples of various procedures such as primary cesarean sections, hysterectomies, gall bladder removals, transurethral resections of the prostate, coronary artery bypass grafts, cardiac catherizations, removals of fatty deposits from the carotial artery, femoral and aortic grafts, total joint replacements, and lamenectomies; and emergency reviews of unplanned returns to the emergency room within 48 hours, and patient deaths in the emergency room or following hospital admission through the emergency room[15].

Comparisons of quality of care across countries are among the least developed concepts in international comparisons. The linkages between quality and outcomes are neither well defined nor easily measurable. Detailed information on quality assurance indicators of the type discussed above is generally not available. Moreover, as discussed below, aggregate mortality and morbidity measures are generally too gross to permit the accurate measurement of quality. Unfortunately, as most comparative studies (including this one) emphasize expenditure and utilisation measures, because these are more readily quantifiable, the quality as well as outcome dimensions are neglected. Death rates, indices of morbidity, or more subtle forms of diminution in quality of life resulting from inadequate or poorly enforced licensing and/or life-safety code standards in hospitals and nursing homes or from inadequately trained medical or para-medical professionals are equally important dimensions of the performance of a health system.

Resource development and distribution policies can also have a substantial impact on physical access to care. Virtually all OECD countries are faced with an aggregate surplus of physicians and acute care hospital beds. In coping with overall surpluses of physicians, most OECD countries are now limiting medical school enrolments, and some are taking steps to encourage physicians to locate in underserved areas by, for example, issuing new billing numbers only for such areas.

Similar arguments can be made for planning activities related to facilities and equipment. The criteria for evaluating and disseminating new technologies are also a critical determinant of cost, quality and access. Some countries have centralised planning, while others rely on local planning. Various formulas and procedures are used to allocate capital, and the financing of and reimbursement for capital costs differ widely, from systems where all capital is allocated and financed centrally to those where authorisation is local and financing/reimbursement is predominantly private.

Legal practices can also have important effects on the delivery system. The extent of malpractice litigation can have substantial effects on health costs not only through the litigation itself but through "defensive medicine" as physicians and hospitals perform extra diagnostic procedures. Anti-trust, medical practice and insurance laws affect the organisation, power and roles of the relevant economic entities (i.e. government, consumers, medical care providers, insurers, employers, trade unions, etc.), determine the permissible delivery arrangements, affect who can practice medicine, and prescribe the interrelationships between public systems and private health insurance. For example, the ability of physicians to organise and negotiate, whether non-physicians can practice medicine as free-standing practitioners, the extent of malpractice suits, and the ability of private insurance companies to sell complementary policies that fill in the cost-sharing and physician "extra charges" can all have significant effects on a health system's performance.

Thus, differences in specific features of health systems can have important effects on utilisation, prices, efficiency, outcomes and quality. Unfortunately, isolating the behavioural impacts of specific systems' features on health systems performance is quite difficult. In the following chapters specific aspects of health systems' performance are analysed, and attempts are made to relate them to particular economic and social characteristics of individual countries.

NOTES AND REFERENCES

1. See Brian Abel-Smith and Alan Maynard, *The Organisation, Financing, and Cost of Health Care in the European Community*, Commission of the European Communities, Brussels, 1979; Gordon McLachlan and Alan Maynard, *The Public/Private Mix for Health: The Relevance and Effects of Change*, Nuffield Provincial Hospital Trust, London, 1982; Jan Blanpain, Bjorn Lindgren, and Simone Sandier, *Comparaisons Internationales des Systemes de Santé*, Centre de Recherche, d'Etude et de Documentation en Economie de la Santé (CREDES), Paris, 1985; *Comparative Tables of the Social Security Schemes in the Member States of the European Communities*, Commission of the European Communities, Luxembourg, 1982; Marshall W. Raffel (ed.), *Comparative Health Systems*, The Pennsylvania

State University Press, University Park and London, 1984; and *Tables of Social Benefit Systems In the Member States of the European Communities, Portugal and Spain (Position at 1st January 1985)*, U.K. Department of Health and Social Security, London, 1985.

2. See Jozef van Langendonck, *Prelude to Harmony on a Community Theme Health Care Insurance Policies in the Six and Britain*, Nuffield Provincial Hospital Trust, London, 1975.

3. See L.A. Aday, R. Anderson, and G.V. Fleming, *Health Care in the United States, Equitable for Whom?*, Sage, Beverley Hills, 1980; and G.H. Mooney, "Equity in Health Care: Confronting the Confusion", *Effective Health Care*, December 1983.

4. For an example of cross-subsidisation, see *Comparaison des Régimes de Sécurité Sociale*, Centre d'Etude des Revenus et des Coûts, Paris, 1983.

5. In less developed countries foreign assistance is another possible financing mechanism.

6. For an analysis of the incidence of financing in Canada, the United States and the United Kingdom see J.W. Hurst, *Financing Health Services in the United States, Canada and Britain*, King Edward's Hospital Fund, London, 1985.

7. For some data on private insurance coverage see *Private Health Insurance*, Comité Européen des Assurances, Paris, 1983.

8. See Peter Townsend and Nick Davidson (eds.), *Inequalities in Health: The Black Report*, Penguin Books Limited., Middlesex, England, 1982; Karen Davis and Kathy Schoen, *Health and the War on Poverty: A Ten Year Appraisal*, The Brookings Institution, Washington, D.C., 1978; and Olle Lundberg, "Class and Health: Comparing Britain and Sweden", *Social Science and Medicine*, Vol. 23, No. 5, 1986.

9. See Brian Abel-Smith, *Cost Containment in Health Care: The Experience of 12 European Countries 1977-83*, EEC, Brussels, 1983; and "Recent Innovations in Social Policy: Secretariat Overview of National Reports", Internal Working Paper, OECD, Paris, 1985.

10. Prior to 1984 the United States Medicare programme reimbursed hospitals on a retrospective basis, whereby hospitals were paid for all reasonable costs incurred in providing medically necessary services to programme beneficiaries. Some private insurers still pay under this approach, while other pay actual billed (not prospectively set) charges.

11. See Uwe E. Reinhardt, "Access, Quality, and Efficiency: Hospitals and Other Institutional Services", in *Health and Pension Policies Under Economic and Demographic Constraints*, OECD, Paris, 1987.

12. See William Glaser, *Paying the Doctor*, Johns Hopkins University Press, Baltimore, 1970.

13. Ambulatory care is not completely closed-ended.

14. The time price to consumers should also be considered.

15. See *Medical Utilisation Review*, McGraw Hill Healthcare Information Center, Washington, D.C., February 6, 1986, pp. 1-2.

Chapter 4

MEASURING THE EFFECTIVENESS
OF HEALTH EXPENDITURES

In order to evaluate the effectiveness of health expenditures in achieving their intended goals of assuring access, quality and efficiency in the production and consumption of health services, the impact of health spending (or spending changes) on "health" must be analysed. This chapter discusses the difficulties in defining and measuring health outcomes. First, the difficulties of defining health status and the problems in isolating the interactive effects of the numerous economic and social forces which influence it are analysed. Second, operational issues in measuring health status and its inherent components of mortality, morbidity and functional disability are discussed. Third, historical data on mortality, morbidity and the costs of illness in OECD countries are presented.

Defining Health

There is no single agreed upon conceptual or operational index of health that:

i)   readily isolates the effects of the multi-dimensional factors affecting health; and
ii) can be used to analyse the plethora of medical, financing, reimbursement and delivery questions facing individuals and governments.

In other words, there is no specific measure to evaluate the multi-billion dollars' worth of health expenditures undertaken annually by OECD countries[1].

It has been increasingly recognised that an individual's health status depends on a variety of factors, including his initial genetic endowment, biomedical knowledge applied through the public health system, the personal service system and lifestyles. Given the number and interactive nature of these medical, social and economic factors, as well as the need to make subjective judgements in their specification, it is not surprising that no single, comprehensive, and universally valid measure exists. Indeed, many of the interesting social policy as well as individual choice questions require information on inputs (e.g. numbers and types of personnel) and

intermediate outputs (e.g. number of hospital days) as well as outcomes.

Health can be defined in either a positive or negative context. The World Health Organisation (WHO) uses a positive definition, "a state of optimal physical, mental and social wellbeing and not merely the absence of disease and infirmity". Most other models or concepts of health are negative in nature. Health is viewed as the absence of illness or, alternatively, illness is perceived as a negative deviation from the norm of "health". In the classic medical model of health status, health is the absence of abnormalities in pathological function caused by specific diseases.

Both the WHO definition and the medical model have been criticised. The WHO concept has been criticised for being too broad and general to be of use in measuring the impacts of specific interventions. The medical model has been criticised for its reliance on medical as opposed to social factors. In particular, it has been criticised for relying on physical disease patterns ("biochemical and morphologic changes within the body which may or may not give rise to symptoms") as opposed to illness effects ("the totality of experience caused by a medical problem: the worries, the fears, the annoyance and the imaginings as well as the physical symptoms")[2]. It has been criticised for neglecting emotional and psychiatric disorders, which are often socially as opposed to pathogenically induced. The medical model has also been criticised for its limited applicability in the preventive and restorative areas.

Attempts have been made to broaden this model to incorporate social factors. This so called "sociological" or "socio-medical" concept of health emphasizes illness as opposed to disease, and explicitly recognises the importance of both physical and socio-physical factors[3].

Increasingly, health and changes in health status are being defined in terms of sets of characteristics which measure individuals' dysfunction (physical and emotional). These characteristics include problems in activities of daily living (e.g. feeding, dressing, mobility, toileting), mental disorders, etc. While, as discussed below, there is currently a great deal of interest in such measures, they are prone to subjective judgements in terms of choice of characteristics, weighting of individual characteristics to develop an individual's index, and aggregating individuals' indices to develop national or sub-national group indices.

Measures of Health Status

Operational measures of health status focus on mortality, morbidity, and dysfunction. Much of the changing emphasis and increased sophistication in such measures has been driven by better data, advances in biomedical and epidemiological knowledge, new social survey techniques, and changing disease and illness patterns.

Operational definitions of health may be aggregate and focus on death, disease and disability in the overall population, or may focus on the disease state and/or levels of functional disability in individuals. The most widely used global measures of health have concentrated on death rates, life expectancy, morbidity rates and various aspects of dysfunction. Crude and age-specific mortality rates, life expectancy by sex and age and age- and sex- specific causes of death, which are reported on the basis of the agreed upon International Classification of Disease (ICD) Codes, are the oldest and most widely available measures of health status. Unfortunately, mortality statistics provide no information about disease incidence or effects (other than the ultimate effect of death). On the other hand, disease incidence statistics provide little information on the physical and emotional impacts of disease on individuals. In fact, there is evidence that increased life expectancy among the elderly is accompanied by increased dysfunction[4]. Moreover, this problem aside, the widely used international measures of mortality and morbidity are generally too aggregate to measure the effects of specific policy interventions, or to differentiate these effects from the numerous economic, social, environmental and other factors that affect morbidity and mortality. Global disability statistics, such as restricted activity days and lost production days, provide only general measures of dysfunction.

With respect to operational measures of health status for individuals, given the generally recognised problems of defining and measuring "good" or "perfect" health and the limitations in conventional mortality and morbidity statistics, researchers have concentrated on developing health status indicators that measure changes in the medical, psychological and social functioning of individuals. Such function or dysfunction is then grouped into different classes or states, and expressed as deviations from the norm of good or perfect health.

Hurst, Culyer, Shanas and Maddox, and Rosser have recently reviewed the available indices[5]. Most of these indices are based on a socio-medical concept of health. They are characterised by two features:

i) a taxonomy of the states of health or alternatively the basic characteristics (or functions) associated with (or with the absence of) good health and;

ii) a scale for attaching values to each state/characteristic as well as, in some cases, a weighting scheme to aggregate individual states/characteristics into a composite index.

The particular states/characteristics generally include functional (social, economic, mental, physical, and activities of daily living) as well as medical indicators.

Subjective valuations of both states/characteristics and aggregation weights are made by patients and/or medical practitioners. Some of the better known indices range from simple measures of number of years of life lost, to the number of life years lost adjusted for quality of life in various states of disability, to restrictions in activities of daily living, to the Rosser and Kind index in which patients, doctors and nurses assess eight states of disability (from no disability to unconsciousness) and four states of distress (none to severe) and rate each cell in the resulting matrix from death [0] to perfect health [1]. In a number of countries researchers have suggested combining an index of this type with years of life lost measures to develop an index of quality-adjusted life years[6].

The Rand Cooperation[7] for use in its Health Insurance Experiment has developed a comprehensive set of health status measures based on four distinct categories: general health, health habits, physiologic health, and the risk of dying from causes related to various risk factors. (The indices were developed from a medical history questionnaire completed by all adults in the experiment and medical screening examinations given at the time of enrolment and exit from the experiment). The specific indicators employed embodied measures of: physical health, mental health, social health, general health perceptions, patient role, weight, overweight and eating habits, diets, medication and psychotropic drugs, types of elective surgery, symptoms in the recent past, chronic illness, stressful life events, patient satisfaction, and other measures.

At present applying these measures for cross-national evaluations of health care policy changes is difficult for several reasons. First, the measures are quite broad. Second, many of these indices, especially those measuring function, are based on subjective valuations, which may differ across countries. Third, the micro data necessary to construct such indices are not readily available in many countries. Fourth, there are the well-known problems for some indices of valuing life. Fifth, the robustness and validity of these measures are still open to question.

Nevertheless, since the following chapters discuss health care expenditures, utilisation, manpower and facility growth from an aggregate perspective, it is useful, despite the limitations cited above, to provide a general picture of mortality and morbidity in OECD countries as well as estimates of the costs of illness.

While such data do not provide precise information on the effects of specific policy interventions, they are useful for describing disease and mortality patterns, and may provide some general insights into resource needs across countries.

Mortality

There have been drastic changes in mortality and morbidity over the past 150 years, resulting from both public health measures and medical interventions. In the mid-19th century death rates, particularly infant mortality rates, were extremely high. The principal causes of disease were microbial infections. From the mid-19th century to the 1930s major reductions in death rates from microbial disease were due largely to increased living standards and public health measures that interrupted the transmission of such microbes through: clean water supplies, sanitation engineering, proper ventilation in home and workplace, and education of new mothers. By the mid-1930s powerful interventions became available (e.g. sulfonamides and chemotherapy for T.B.). By the 1950s, these measures as well as increased standards of living resulted in substantial increases in life expectancy and changes in the causes of death. Infectious diseases have become a minor problem, and with increased life expectancy chronic diseases have now become the most prevalent causes of death in OECD countries. In other words, the developed countries have undergone an "Epidemiologic Transition" in which high infant mortality rates caused by infectious diseases have been substantially reduced, while most deaths now occur in the middle or later years as a result of chronic diseases[8].

In addition, some now argue that 80 per cent of the years of life lost to non-traumatic premature deaths have been eliminated, and that there is little that conventional medical interventions can do to extend these biologically defined limits on life. In other words, the mortality and morbidity curves of individuals have become increasingly "rectangularised", that is, individuals tend to live their full biological lives without the interruption of premature death. There is, however, a debate about the health status of these individuals[9].

By some estimates 80 per cent of all deaths and an even greater percentage of total disability are now due to chronic illness. Little is known about the causes of these chronic diseases. It is unlikely that medical breakthroughs will cure chronic disease, since much of it is simply due to the normal ageing process and deterioration in the functioning capacity of body organs. Prevention of chronic disease is in its infancy. The greatest potential for increasing life expectancy would result from a better understanding of the ageing process and its retardation through breakthroughs in molecular biology[10].

Table 8 provides historical information on infant mortality rates for males and females from 1900 to the early 1980s for the OECD countries. Infant mortality rates both for males and for females declined by over 90 per cent between 1900 and the early 1980s. Infant deaths per 1 000 births for males declined from an OECD average (16 countries) of 144 in 1900, to 83 in 1930, to 45 in 1950 and to 11 in the 1980s. For females the rates declined from 122 in 1900, to 68 in 1930, to 37 in 1950 and to 9 in the 1980s. The largest absolute declines occurred in the 1900-1950 period, largely as a result of public health measures, improved education, and increased standards of living. More recently, the implementation and diffusion of effective medical interventions made widely accessible through public and private health financing programmes, prevention and education programmes targeted to vulnerable groups, and new diagnostic and therapeutic technologies for pregnant women and newborns (e.g. ultra sound, amniosynthesis, neo-natal intensive care) resulted in smaller, yet significant, declines in infant death rates to levels that are so low that further appreciable reductions are considered unlikely.

The variations in infant death rates across OECD countries have also narrowed. In 1900 death rates for males ranged from 82 per 1 000 births in Norway to 232 in Austria with a 16-country OECD average of 144, while for females the rates ranged from 67 in Norway to 191 in Spain with an average of 122. By the early 1980s the distribution (23 countries) had become increasingly condensed, ranging for males from 6.5 in Finland to 22.1 in Portugal with an average of less than 12, while female death rates ranged from 5.6 in Japan to 17.3 in Portugal with an average of 9.

Also, the data indicate that the gap between male and female infant death rates has widened. For the 16 countries for which consistent data are available for the entire time period, male infant mortality rates were 18 per cent higher than female rates in 1900, 22 per cent in 1930, and 24 per cent in 1950 and in the early 1980s. The same trend is found for the average infant death rates based on information for all countries.

Along with drastic declines in infant death rates, there have also been significant increases in life expectancy at all ages. Tables 9, 10 and 11 display life expectancy at birth, age 40 and age 65 for males and females in 1900, 1930, 1950 and the early 1980s for the OECD countries. Tables 12, 13 and 14 display the respective increases in terms of the absolute total and average annual gains in additional years of life, as well as the percentage increase over the period. Life expectancy at birth has increased for males from an average (19 countries) of 48.0 years in 1900, to 57.1 years in 1930, to 65.4 years in 1950 and to 71.7 years in the early 1980s. For the entire 1900-1980s period male life expectancy at birth increased by 23.7 years (52 per cent), and 0.29 year of increase per year. The largest increases occurred in the 1900-1950 period. Average annual increases in years of life for males at birth increased at .30 year between 1900-1930 and .42 year between 1930-1950, compared to .20 year between 1950-1980s.

Table 8

INFANT DEATH RATES BY SEX
(Deaths of infants per 1 000 live births)

	Circa	Males				Females			
		1900	1930	1950	1980s	1900	1930	1950	1980s
Australia		95.1	45.4	32.0	10.5 (83)	79.5	36.4	25.2	8.7
Austria		232.3	115.4	75.2	13.4 (83)	189.9	92.5	58.4	10.0
Belgium			100.8	64.0	13.4 (79)		78.6	49.3	11.2
Canada			87.0	43.3	10.4 (82)		69.3	34.2	7.8
Denmark		130.7	91.3	45.3	9.5 (82)	104.1	71.1	34.7	6.9
Finland		134.5	99.8	43.6	6.5 (83)	113.1	82.8	33.6	5.8
France		163.3	90.2	52.1	11.2 (81)	136.5	71.6	40.2	8.2
Germany		202.3	85.4	61.8	10.6 (84)	170.5	68.4	49.1	8.9
Greece			95.1	65.0	16.4 (82)		93.1	58.7	13.6
Iceland		120.8	56.6	33.4	7.8 (82)	104.6	49.2	28.6	6.2
Ireland			77.2	49.5	11.2 (81)		63.5	39.0	9.3
Italy		167.7	115.3	67.5	17.1 (79)	152.1	102.3	58.5	13.8
Japan		156.9	140.1	65.8	6.6 (84)	140.9	124.1	57.6	5.6
Luxembourg				48.0	12.3 (82)			43.0	12.9
Netherlands		140.5	65.3	27.8	9.2 (83)	117.7	50.6	21.5	7.5
New Zealand		83.1	38.6	25.0	14.1 (83)	68.5	25.5	20.0	11.6
Norway		81.5	55.1	34.2	8.7 (83)	66.8	44.1	25.7	7.0
Portugal				104.6	22.1 (82)			92.5	17.3
Spain		210.5	123.6	68.7	16.1 (79)	190.8	109.0	59.1	12.6
Sweden		92.6	64.7	26.6	7.1 (82)	76.0	50.5	20.5	6.5
Switzerland			56.2	35.9	8.0 (84)		44.1	27.7	6.2
Turkey									
United Kingdom[a]		160.0	71.9	32.7	12.2 (82)	131.0	54.6	25.1	9.4
United States		135.7	65.6	33.4	12.8 (82)	112.7	52.7	25.9	10.2
Mean*		144.2	82.8	45.3	10.8	122.1	67.8	36.5	8.7
High-Low*		150.8	101.5	50.2	10.6	124.0	98.6	39.1	8.2
Standard Deviation*		45.1	29.8	17.3	3.3	39.8	87.8	15.1	2.5
Mean - All Countries		144.2	82.9	49.4	11.6	122.1	68.3	40.4	9.4

Notes: a) England and Wales.
  * Excludes Belgium, Canada, Greece, Ireland, Luxembourg, Portugal, Switzerland and Turkey.

Sources: Demographic Yearbook, 1957, 1961, United Nations, New York, 1957, 1961.
World Health Statistics, 1983, 1984, 1985, World Health Organisation, Geneva, 1983, 1984, 1985. Complemented by data from Statistical Yearbook of Greece (1961), Spain (1985), Luxembourg (1984/85), Italy (1952), and the United Kingdom (1986).
The Japanese Ministry of Health and Welfare, "Outline of Recent Japanese Policy on Health: The Background and Measures for Reform", Health and Pension Policies Under Economic and Demographic Constraints, OECD, Paris, 1987.

Similar patterns are found for increases in life expectancy at birth for females. Female life expectancy at birth increased from 50.6 years in 1900, to 60.2 in 1930, to 69.6 in 1950 and to 78.5 in the 1980s. For the entire 1900-1980s period female life expectancy at birth increased by 27.9 years (57 per cent), and 0.34 year of increase per year. Average annual increases in years of life were 0.32 between 1900-1930, 0.47 between 1930-1950, compared to 0.28 between 1950-1980s. Gains in life expectancy at birth for females have exceeded those for males in every time period, and for the overall period female life expectancy at birth increased by 27.9 years (57 per cent), compared to 23.7 years (52 per cent) for males. As discussed below, much of this differential increase is due to differential reductions in death rates in the higher age ranges.

Also of interest is the large reduction in differences in life expectancy at birth among (the 19) countries. In 1900 the differences in life expectancy between the country with the highest life expectancy and that with the lowest was 24.2 years for males and 24.9 years for females. These differences have progressively and consistently diminished to 5.3 years for males and 5.0 years

for females in the early 1980s. Analogously, the distributions of life expectancies at birth around the mean have become significantly more concentrated, as evinced by coefficients of variation in 1900 of 0.12 for both males and females, compared to coefficients of 0.02 for both males and females in the early 1980s. In fact, in the early 1980s 23 of the 24 OECD countries have both male and female life expectancies at birth that fall within a band of plus or minus 3.1 years around the OECD average.

Life expectancies at age 40 and age 65 have also increased significantly, although the sizes, timing and differential impacts by sex of the increases are somewhat different. For males life expectancy at age 40 has increased from 27.9 years in 1900, to 29.9 years in 1930, to 32 years in 1950 and to 33.8 years in 1980. For the entire 80-year period life expectancy has increased by 5.8 years (21.4 per cent), and .07 year per year. The increases were spread over all three time periods, but the largest increases took place between 1930 and 1950.

A slightly different picture emerges for females. Life expectancy at age 40 has increased from 30 years in 1900, to 32 years in 1930, to 35.1 years in 1950 and to

Table 9

LIFE EXPECTANCY AT BIRTH

			Males				Females	
	Circa 1900	1930	1950	1980s	1900	1930	1950	1980s
Australia	55.2	63.5	66.5	72.2 (83)	58.8	67.1	71.7	79.0
Austria	39.1	54.5	62.2	69.5 (83)	41.1	58.5	67.3	76.6
Belgium	45.4	56.0	63.8	69.9 (79)	48.8	59.8	69.0	76.6
Canada		60.0	66.3	72.0 (82)		62.1	70.5	79.0
Denmark	52.9	60.9	69.2	71.8 (82)	56.2	62.6	71.7	77.9
Finland	45.3	50.7	61.4	70.2 (83)	48.1	55.1	68.1	78.5
France	45.3	54.3	63.9	70.9 (81)	48.7	59.0	69.7	79.1
Germany	44.8	59.9	64.4	71.3 (84)	48.3	62.8	68.3	78.1
Greece		49.1	63.4	73.6 (82)		50.9	66.6	78.3
Iceland	48.3	56.2	68.7	73.4 (83)	53.1	61.0	73.6	80.6
Ireland	49.3	57.4	64.5	70.1 (81)	49.6	57.9	67.1	75.8
Italy	44.2	53.8	64.3	71.0 (80)	44.8	56.0	67.9	77.7
Japan	44.0	44.8	57.5	74.8 (84)	44.8	46.5	60.8	80.7
Luxembourg			61.7	68.9 (82)			65.7	76.0
Netherlands	51.0	61.9	70.5	73.0 (83)	53.7	63.5	72.8	79.8
New Zealand	58.1	65.0	67.4	70.8 (83)	60.6	67.9	71.1	77.0
Norway	54.8	61.0	70.0	72.8 (83)	57.7	63.8	73.4	79.8
Portugal			56.1	69.1 (82)			61.3	76.1
Spain	33.9	48.4	59.8	71.8 (79)	35.7	51.6	64.3	78.0
Sweden	54.5	61.0	69.9	73.5 (82)	57.0	63.2	72.4	79.6
Switzerland	49.3	59.2	66.9	73.8 (84)	52.2	63.1	71.3	80.8
Turkey				58.3 a				62.8
United Kingdom[b]	48.5	58.8	66.5	71.3 (82)	52.4	62.9	71.3	77.3
United States	47.9	57.7	65.6	70.9 (82)	50.7	61.0	71.2	78.4
Mean*	48.0	57.1	65.4	71.7	50.6	60.2	69.6	78.5
High-Low*	24.2	20.2	13.0	5.3	24.9	21.4	12.8	5.0
Standard Deviation*	5.9	5.2	3.6	1.5	6.3	5.2	3.3	1.5
Mean - All Countries	48.0	56.9	64.8	71.0	50.6	59.8	69.0	77.7

Notes: a) 1976-80; b) England and Wales; * Excludes Canada, Greece, Luxembourg, Portugal and Turkey.

Sources: Demographic Yearbook, 1957, 1983. United Nations, New York, 1957, 1985.
World Health Statistics Annual, 1983, 1984, 1985. World Health Organisation, Geneva, 1983, 1984, 1985.
Economic Survey of Europe in 1974 Part II, Post-War Demographic Trends In Europe and the Outlook Until the Year 2000. United Nations, New York, 1975.

39.4 years in 1980. For the entire 80-year period life expectancy has increased by 9.4 years (versus 5.8 for males), 32 per cent (versus 21 per cent for males) and 0.12 year per year. The largest increases in life expectancy for females took place between 1930-1980, when the annual gain in years was more than double the 1900-1930 increases.

As in the case of life expectancy at birth, the distributions of life expectancy at age 40 have become somewhat more condensed, as shown by reductions in the coefficients of variation from about .07 in 1900 to .04 in 1980. Interestingly, there was less variability in the distribution of life expectancy at age 40 than at birth in 1900, and relatively more variability in 1980.

Life expectancy at age 65 has also progressively increased but the impact has been greater for women than for men. Life expectancy at age 65 for men has increased from 11.1 years in 1900, to 11.9 years in 1930, to 12.7 years in 1950 and to 14 years in the early 1980s. Over the entire 1900-1980s period life expectancy at age 65 for males increased by 3.0 years, 28 per cent and by .04 year per year. The largest annual increases took place between 1930-1980s.

For females life expectancy at 65 has increased from 11.9 years in 1900, to 13 years in 1930, to 14.3 years in 1950 and to 18 years in the early 1980s. For the entire period life expectancy for females increased by 6.1 years (53 per cent), and by .08 year per year. These increases in female life expectancy were more than double the increases for males, and have resulted in sizeable and increasing differences between males and females in life expectancy at birth. The major annual increases in life expectancy at 65 for females took place between 1950-1980s, when the average annual gain in years was almost double the 1930-1950 period and over three times the 1900-1930 increase. There is, however, currently relatively more variability across countries in life expectancy at 65, as evinced by coefficients of variation of .06 compared to .04 for life expectancy at 40 and .02 for life expectancy at birth, although the variability has been reduced since 1900 (coefficient of variation of .10).

As discussed above, differences in life expectancy between males and females have increased substantially. In 1900 life expectancy for females at birth exceeded that of males by 2.6 years, in 1930 by 3.1

Table 10

LIFE EXPECTANCY AT AGE 40

	Circa	Males				Females			
		1900	1930	1950	1980	1900	1930	1950	1980
Australia		28.6	31.1	31.4	33.9	31.5	34.0	35.4	39.9
Austria		25.8	28.7	30.9	32.5	27.1	31.1	34.5	38.3
Belgium		26.7	29.5	31.1	32.0	29.5	31.8	34.8	37.5
Canada			32.0	32.5	34.0		33.0	35.6	41.0
Denmark		29.4	32.0	34.1	33.9	31.7	32.4	35.3	39.2
Finland		27.4	27.6	28.9	31.8	29.9	31.0	34.0	39.0
France		26.7	27.6	30.8	33.2	29.1	31.4	35.4	40.2
Germany		26.7	30.8	32.3	32.9	29.2	32.3	34.6	38.6
Greece			29.8	35.0	36.4		32.4	37.5	40.1
Iceland		27.2	30.5	34.2	36.5	31.8	33.7	37.4	41.6
Ireland		31.0	30.4	31.6	32.0	30.9	30.8	33.3	36.2
Italy		28.2	30.4	33.1	33.7	29.2	32.1	35.8	39.5
Japan		26.0	25.7	29.1	35.9	28.2	29.0	32.2	40.7
Luxembourg				30.3	31.3			33.4	37.1
Netherlands		29.5	32.1	34.9	34.7	30.8	32.5	36.2	40.7
New Zealand		30.1	32.1	32.5	33.1	32.0	33.8	35.4	38.5
Norway		31.5	32.4	35.1	34.7	32.9	34.0	37.1	40.4
Portugal				30.7	32.0			34.9	38.0
Spain		25.0	27.5	30.4	34.5	26.4	30.4	33.9	39.6
Sweden		30.1	32.3	34.1	34.9	32.5	33.4	35.6	40.4
Switzerland		26.0	28.6	32.3	35.1	28.4	31.4	35.5	40.7
Turkey									
United Kingdom a		27.0	29.6	31.3	32.7	29.4	32.6	35.4	38.2
United States		27.7	28.7	30.9	33.3	29.1	30.1	35.2	39.8
Mean*		27.9	29.9	32.0	33.8	30.0	32.0	35.1	39.4
High-Low*		6.5	6.7	6.2	4.7	6.5	5.0	5.2	5.4
Standard Deviation*		1.9	1.9	1.8	1.3	1.8	1.4	1.2	1.3
Mean - All Countries		27.9	30.0	32.0	33.7	30.0	32.0	35.1	39.3

Notes: a) England and Wales. * Excludes Canada, Greece, Luxembourg, Portugal and Turkey.

Sources: Measuring Health Care 1960-1983, OECD, Paris, 1985, Table F.1.
Demographic Yearbook, 1957, United Nations, New York, 1957.

Table 11

LIFE EXPECTANCY AT AGE 65

	Circa	Males				Females			
		1900	1930	1950	1980s	1900	1930	1950	1980s
Australia		11.3	12.4	12.2	14.3 (83)	12.9	14.2	14.4	18.6
Austria		10.1	11.2	12.0	13.1 (83)	10.2	12.1	13.6	16.6
Belgium		10.6	11.4	12.3	12.9 (79)	11.6	12.6	13.9	16.9
Canada			13.0	13.3	14.5 (82)		13.7	15.0	18.7
Denmark		11.9	12.6	13.9	14.0 (82)	13.0	12.9	14.6	18.1
Finland		10.8	11.3	11.0	13.0 (83)	11.9	12.5	13.1	17.5
France		10.5	10.9	11.9	14.3 (81)	11.5	12.6	14.4	18.7
Germany		10.4	11.9	12.8	13.6 (84)	11.1	12.6	13.7	17.6
Greece			13.1	13.0	15.4 (82)		14.1	14.4	17.6
Iceland		11.7	13.0	14.7	15.3 (83)	13.4	14.9	15.9	19.4
Ireland		10.8	12.8	12.1	12.5 (81)	10.6	13.4	13.3	15.8
Italy		10.7	11.9	12.6	13.8 (80)	10.8	12.7	13.7	17.4
Japan		10.1	9.6	11.2	15.7 (84)	11.4	11.6	13.2	19.3
Luxembourg				11.9	13.0 (82)			13.4	16.6
Netherlands		11.6	12.5	14.1	14.0 (83)	12.3	13.0	14.7	19.0
New Zealand		12.2	12.9	12.9	13.6 (83)	13.3	13.8	14.8	17.5
Norway		13.5	13.7	14.9	14.5 (83)	14.4	14.6	16.0	18.7
Portugal				11.9	13.7 (82)			14.0	16.8
Spain		9.0	10.4	12.0	14.4 (79)	9.2	11.5	14.0	17.5
Sweden		12.8	13.2	13.5	14.6 (82)	13.7	13.9	14.3	18.2
Switzerland		10.1	11.0	12.4	15.5 (84)	10.7	12.1	14.0	19.8
Turkey									
United Kingdom a		10.8	11.3	12.0	13.1 (82)	12.0	13.1	14.4	17.2
United States		11.5	11.7	12.7	14.6 (82)	12.2	12.8	15.0	19.1
Mean*		11.1	11.9	12.7	14.0	11.9	13.0	14.3	18.0
High-Low*		4.5	4.1	3.9	3.2	5.2	3.4	2.9	4.0
Standard Deviation*		1.1	1.1	1.1	0.9	1.3	0.9	0.8	1.1
Mean - All Countries		11.1	12.0	12.7	14.0	11.9	13.1	14.3	17.9

Notes: a) England and Wales; * Excludes Canada, Greece, Luxembourg, Portugal and Turkey.

Sources: Demographic Yearbook, 1957, 1983, United Nations, New York, 1957, 1985.
World Health Statistics Annual, 1983, 1984, 1985, World Health Organisation, Geneva 1983, 1984, 1985.
Economic Survey of Europe in 1974 Part II, Post War Demographic Trends in Europe and the Outlook Until the Year 2000, United Nations, New York, 1975.
Statistical Yearbook of Greece, 1981.

Table 12

GAIN IN YEARS FROM CHANGES OF LIFE EXPECTANCY AT BIRTH

		1900 - 1930			1930 - 1950			1950 - 1980s			1900-1980s		
		Number of years	% increase	Annual increase in years	Number of years	% increase	Annual increase in years	Number of years	% increase	Annual increase in years	Number of years	% increase	Annual increase in years
Australia	M	8.300	15.036	0.277	3.000	4.724	0.150	5.700	8.571	0.173	17.000	30.797	0.205
	F	8.300	14.116	0.277	4.600	6.855	0.230	7.300	10.181	0.221	20.200	34.354	0.243
Austria	M	15.400	39.386	0.513	7.700	14.128	0.385	7.300	11.736	0.221	30.400	77.749	0.366
	F	17.400	42.336	0.580	8.800	15.043	0.440	9.300	13.819	0.282	35.500	86.375	0.428
Belgium	M	10.600	23.348	0.353	7.800	13.929	0.390	6.100	9.561	0.210	24.500	53.965	0.310
	F	11.000	22.541	0.367	9.200	15.385	0.460	7.600	11.014	0.262	27.800	56.967	0.352
Canada	M	..	..	..	6.300	10.500	0.315	5.700	8.597	0.178	..	..	..
	F	..	..	..	8.400	13.527	0.420	8.500	12.057	0.265	..	..	..
Denmark	M	8.000	15.123	0.267	8.300	13.629	0.415	2.600	3.757	0.081	18.900	35.728	0.230
	F	6.400	11.388	0.213	9.100	14.537	0.455	6.200	8.647	0.194	21.700	38.612	0.265
Finland	M	5.400	11.921	0.180	10.700	21.105	0.535	8.800	14.332	0.267	24.900	54.967	0.300
	F	7.000	14.553	0.233	13.000	23.593	0.650	10.400	15.272	0.315	30.400	63.202	0.366
France	M	9.000	19.868	0.300	9.600	17.680	0.480	7.000	10.955	0.226	25.600	56.512	0.316
	F	10.300	21.150	0.343	10.700	18.136	0.535	9.400	13.486	0.303	30.400	62.423	0.375
Germany	M	15.100	33.705	0.503	4.500	7.513	0.225	6.900	10.714	0.203	26.500	59.152	0.315
	F	14.500	30.021	0.483	5.500	8.758	0.275	9.800	14.348	0.288	29.800	61.698	0.355
Greece	M	..	..	..	14.300	29.124	0.715	10.200	16.090	0.319	..	..	..
	F	..	..	..	15.700	30.845	0.785	11.700	17.568	0.366	..	..	..
Iceland	M	7.900	16.356	0.263	12.500	22.242	0.625	4.700	6.841	0.142	25.100	51.967	0.302
	F	7.900	14.878	0.263	12.600	20.656	0.630	7.000	9.511	0.212	27.500	51.789	0.331
Ireland	M	8.100	16.430	0.270	7.100	12.369	0.355	5.600	8.682	0.181	20.800	42.191	0.257
	F	8.300	16.734	0.277	9.200	15.889	0.460	8.700	12.966	0.281	26.200	52.823	0.323
Italy	M	9.600	21.719	0.320	10.500	19.517	0.525	6.700	10.420	0.223	26.800	60.633	0.335
	F	11.200	25.000	0.373	11.900	21.250	0.595	9.800	14.433	0.327	32.900	73.438	0.411
Japan	M	0.800	1.818	0.027	12.700	28.348	0.635	17.300	30.087	0.509	30.800	70.000	0.367
	F	1.700	3.795	0.057	14.300	30.753	0.715	19.900	32.730	0.585	35.900	80.134	0.427
Luxembourg	M	..	..	..	..	..	..	7.200	11.669	0.225	..	..	..
	F	..	..	..	..	..	..	10.300	15.677	0.322	..	..	..
Netherlands	M	10.900	21.373	0.363	8.600	13.893	0.430	2.500	3.546	0.076	22.000	43.137	0.265
	F	9.800	18.250	0.327	9.300	14.646	0.465	7.000	9.615	0.212	26.100	48.603	0.314
New Zealand	M	6.900	11.876	0.230	2.400	3.692	0.120	3.400	5.045	0.103	12.700	21.859	0.153
	F	7.300	12.046	0.243	3.200	4.713	0.160	5.900	8.298	0.179	16.400	27.063	0.198
Norway	M	6.200	11.314	0.207	9.000	14.754	0.450	2.800	4.000	0.085	18.000	32.847	0.217
	F	6.100	10.572	0.203	9.600	15.047	0.480	6.400	8.719	0.194	22.100	38.302	0.266
Portugal	M	..	..	..	..	..	..	13.000	23.173	0.406	..	..	..
	F	..	..	..	..	..	..	14.800	24.140	0.463	..	..	..
Spain	M	14.500	42.773	0.483	11.400	23.554	0.570	12.000	20.067	0.414	37.900	111.799	0.480
	F	15.900	44.538	0.530	12.700	24.612	0.635	13.700	21.306	0.472	42.300	118.487	0.535
Sweden	M	6.500	11.927	0.217	8.900	14.590	0.445	3.600	5.150	0.112	19.000	34.862	0.232
	F	6.200	10.877	0.207	9.200	14.557	0.460	7.200	9.945	0.225	22.600	39.649	0.276
Switzerland	M	9.900	20.081	0.330	7.700	13.007	0.385	6.900	10.314	0.203	24.500	49.696	0.292
	F	10.900	20.881	0.363	8.200	12.995	0.410	9.500	13.324	0.279	28.600	54.789	0.340
United Kingdom	M	10.300	21.237	0.343	7.700	13.095	0.385	4.800	7.218	0.150	22.800	47.010	0.278
	F	10.500	20.038	0.350	8.400	13.355	0.420	6.000	8.415	0.188	24.900	47.519	0.304
United States	M	9.800	20.459	0.327	7.900	13.692	0.395	5.300	8.079	0.166	23.000	48.017	0.280
	F	10.300	20.316	0.343	10.200	16.721	0.510	7.200	10.112	0.225	27.700	54.635	0.338
Average	M	9.116	19.776	0.304	8.316	15.024	0.416	6.316	9.951	0.197	23.747	51.731	0.289
	F	9.526	19.686	0.317	9.458	16.184	0.473	8.858	12.955	0.276	27.842	57.414	0.339
Range	M	14.600	40.955	0.487	10.300	24.656	0.515	14.800	26.541	0.433	25.200	89.940	0.327
	F	15.700	40.743	0.523	11.100	26.040	0.555	14.000	24.430	0.406	25.900	91.425	0.338
Standard Deviation	M	3.496	9.933	0.117	2.789	6.145	0.139	3.535	6.317	0.109	5.670	20.034	0.072
	F	3.706	10.299	0.124	2.852	6.195	0.143	3.307	5.783	0.102	6.136	21.277	0.078

Source: Table 9.

Table 13

GAIN IN YEARS FROM CHANGES OF LIFE EXPECTANCY AT AGE 40

		1900 - 1930			1930 - 1950			1950 - 1980			1900-1980		
		Number of years	% increase	Annual increase in years	Number of years	% increase	Annual increase in years	Number of years	% increase	Annual increase in years	Number of years	% increase	Annual increase in years
Australia	M	2.500	8.741	0.083	0.300	0.965	0.015	2.500	7.962	0.083	5.300	18.531	0.066
	F	2.500	7.937	0.083	1.400	4.118	0.070	4.500	12.712	0.150	8.400	26.667	0.105
Austria	M	2.900	11.240	0.097	2.200	7.666	0.110	1.600	5.178	0.053	6.700	25.969	0.084
	F	4.000	14.760	0.133	3.400	10.932	0.170	3.800	11.014	0.127	11.200	41.328	0.140
Belgium	M	2.800	10.487	0.093	1.600	5.424	0.080	0.900	2.894	0.030	5.300	19.850	0.066
	F	2.300	7.797	0.077	3.000	9.434	0.150	2.700	7.759	0.090	8.000	27.119	0.100
Canada	M	..	..	..	0.500	1.563	0.025	1.500	4.615	0.050	..	..	..
	F	..	..	..	2.600	7.879	0.130	5.400	15.169	0.180	..	..	..
Denmark	M	2.600	8.844	0.087	2.100	6.562	0.105	-0.200	-0.587	-0.007	4.500	15.306	0.056
	F	0.700	2.208	0.023	2.900	8.951	0.145	3.900	11.048	0.130	7.500	23.659	0.094
Finland	M	0.200	0.730	0.007	1.300	4.710	0.065	2.900	10.035	0.097	4.400	16.058	0.055
	F	1.100	3.679	0.037	3.000	9.677	0.150	5.000	14.706	0.167	9.100	30.435	0.114
France	M	0.900	3.371	0.030	3.200	11.594	0.160	2.400	7.792	0.080	6.500	24.345	0.081
	F	2.300	7.904	0.077	4.000	12.739	0.200	4.800	13.559	0.160	11.100	38.144	0.139
Germany	M	4.100	15.356	0.137	1.500	4.870	0.075	0.600	1.858	0.020	6.200	23.221	0.078
	F	3.100	10.616	0.103	2.300	7.121	0.115	4.000	11.561	0.133	9.400	32.192	0.118
Greece	M	..	..	..	5.200	17.450	0.260	1.400	4.000	0.047	..	..	..
	F	..	..	..	5.100	15.740	0.255	2.600	6.933	0.087	..	..	..
Iceland	M	3.300	12.132	0.110	3.700	12.131	0.185	2.300	6.725	0.077	9.300	34.191	0.116
	F	1.900	5.975	0.063	3.700	10.979	0.185	4.200	11.230	0.140	9.800	30.818	0.122
Ireland	M	-0.600	-1.935	-0.020	1.200	3.947	0.060	0.400	1.266	0.013	1.000	3.226	0.012
	F	-0.100	-0.324	-0.003	2.500	8.117	0.125	2.900	8.709	0.097	5.300	17.152	0.066
Italy	M	2.200	7.801	0.073	2.700	8.882	0.135	0.600	1.813	0.020	5.500	19.504	0.069
	F	2.900	9.932	0.097	3.700	11.526	0.185	3.700	10.335	0.123	10.300	35.274	0.129
Japan	M	-0.300	-1.154	-0.010	3.400	13.230	0.170	6.800	23.368	0.227	9.900	38.077	0.124
	F	0.800	2.837	0.027	3.200	11.034	0.160	8.500	26.398	0.283	12.500	44.326	0.156
Luxembourg	M	..	..	..	..	..	..	1.000	3.300	0.033	..	..	..
	F	..	..	..	..	..	..	3.700	11.078	0.123	..	..	..
Netherlands	M	2.600	8.814	0.087	2.800	8.723	0.140	-0.200	-0.573	-0.007	5.200	17.627	0.065
	F	1.700	5.519	0.057	3.700	11.385	0.185	4.500	12.431	0.150	9.900	32.143	0.124
New Zealand	M	2.000	6.645	0.067	0.400	1.246	0.020	0.600	1.846	0.020	3.000	9.967	0.038
	F	1.800	5.625	0.060	1.600	4.734	0.080	3.100	8.757	0.103	6.500	20.312	0.081
Norway	M	0.900	2.857	0.030	2.700	8.333	0.135	-0.400	-1.140	-0.013	3.200	10.159	0.040
	F	1.100	3.343	0.037	3.100	9.118	0.155	3.300	8.895	0.110	7.500	22.796	0.094
Portugal	M	..	..	..	..	..	..	1.300	4.235	0.043	..	..	..
	F	..	..	..	..	..	..	3.100	8.883	0.103	..	..	..
Spain	M	2.500	10.000	0.083	2.900	10.545	0.145	4.100	13.487	0.137	9.500	38.000	0.119
	F	4.000	15.152	0.133	3.500	11.513	0.175	5.700	16.814	0.190	13.200	50.000	0.165
Sweden	M	2.200	7.309	0.073	1.800	5.573	0.090	0.800	2.346	0.027	4.800	15.947	0.060
	F	0.900	2.769	0.030	2.200	6.587	0.110	4.800	13.483	0.160	7.900	24.308	0.099
Switzerland	M	2.600	10.000	0.087	3.700	12.937	0.185	2.800	8.669	0.093	9.100	35.000	0.114
	F	3.000	10.563	0.100	4.100	13.057	0.205	5.200	14.648	0.173	12.300	43.310	0.154
United Kingdom	M	2.600	9.630	0.087	1.700	5.743	0.085	1.400	4.473	0.047	5.700	21.111	0.071
	F	3.200	10.884	0.107	2.800	8.589	0.140	2.800	7.910	0.093	8.800	29.932	0.110
United States	M	1.000	3.610	0.033	2.200	7.666	0.110	2.400	7.767	0.080	5.600	20.217	0.070
	F	1.000	3.436	0.033	5.100	16.944	0.255	4.600	13.068	0.153	10.700	36.770	0.134
Average	M	1.947	7.077	0.065	2.179	7.407	0.109	1.700	5.536	0.057	5.826	21.385	0.073
	F	2.010	6.874	0.067	3.116	9.818	0.156	4.316	12.370	0.144	9.442	31.931	0.118
Range	M	4.700	17.291	0.157	3.400	12.265	0.170	7.200	24.507	0.240	8.900	34.851	0.111
	F	4.100	15.475	0.136	3.700	12.826	0.185	5.800	18.639	0.193	7.900	32.848	0.099
Standard Deviation	M	1.252	4.650	0.042	1.006	3.613	0.050	1.746	5.895	0.058	2.338	9.568	0.029
	F	1.164	4.296	0.038	0.890	3.018	0.044	1.326	4.215	0.044	2.102	8.797	0.026

Source: Table 10.

40

Table 14

GAIN IN YEARS FROM CHANGES OF LIFE EXPECTANCY AT AGE 65

		1900 - 1930			1930 - 1950			1950 - 1980s			1900 - 1980s		
		Number of years	% increase	Annual increase in years	Number of years	% increase	Annual increase in years	Number of years	% increase	Annual increase in years	Number of years	% increase	Annual increase in years
Australia	M	1.100	9.735	0.037	-0.200	-1.613	-0.010	2.100	17.213	0.064	3.000	26.549	0.036
	F	1.300	10.078	0.043	0.200	1.408	0.010	4.200	29.167	0.127	5.700	44.186	0.069
Austria	M	1.100	10.891	0.037	0.800	7.143	0.040	1.100	9.167	0.033	3.000	29.703	0.036
	F	1.900	18.627	0.063	1.500	12.397	0.075	3.000	22.059	0.091	6.400	62.745	0.077
Belgium	M	0.800	7.547	0.027	0.900	7.895	0.045	0.600	4.878	0.021	2.300	21.698	0.029
	F	1.000	8.621	0.033	1.300	10.317	0.065	3.000	21.583	0.103	5.300	45.690	0.067
Canada	M	..	..	..	0.300	2.310	0.015	1.200	9.023	0.038	..	..	..
	F	..	..	..	1.300	9.489	0.065	3.700	24.667	0.116	..	..	..
Denmark	M	0.700	5.882	0.023	1.300	10.317	0.065	0.100	0.719	0.003	2.100	17.647	0.026
	F	-0.100	-0.769	-0.003	1.700	13.178	0.085	3.500	23.973	0.109	5.100	39.231	0.062
Finland	M	0.500	4.630	0.017	-0.300	-2.655	-0.015	2.000	18.182	0.061	2.200	20.370	0.027
	F	0.600	5.042	0.020	0.600	4.800	0.030	4.400	33.588	0.133	5.600	47.059	0.067
France	M	0.400	3.810	0.013	1.000	9.174	0.050	2.400	20.168	0.077	3.800	36.190	0.047
	F	1.100	9.565	0.037	1.800	14.286	0.090	4.300	29.861	0.139	7.200	62.609	0.089
Germany	M	1.500	14.423	0.050	0.900	7.563	0.045	0.800	6.250	0.024	3.200	30.769	0.038
	F	1.500	13.514	0.050	1.100	8.730	0.055	3.900	28.467	0.115	6.500	58.559	0.077
Greece	M	..	..	..	-0.100	-0.763	-0.005	2.400	18.460	0.075	..	..	..
	F	..	..	..	0.300	2.128	0.015	3.200	22.220	0.100	..	..	..
Iceland	M	1.300	11.111	0.043	1.700	13.077	0.085	0.600	4.082	0.018	3.600	30.769	0.043
	F	1.500	11.194	0.050	1.000	6.711	0.050	3.500	22.013	0.106	6.000	44.776	0.072
Ireland	M	2.000	18.519	0.067	-0.700	-5.469	-0.035	0.400	3.306	0.013	1.700	15.741	0.021
	F	2.800	26.415	0.093	-0.100	-0.746	-0.005	2.500	18.797	0.081	5.200	49.057	0.064
Italy	M	1.200	11.215	0.040	0.700	5.882	0.035	1.200	9.524	0.040	3.100	28.972	0.039
	F	1.900	17.593	0.063	1.000	7.874	0.050	3.700	27.007	0.123	6.600	61.111	0.082
Japan	M	-0.500	-4.950	-0.017	1.600	16.667	0.080	4.500	40.179	0.132	5.600	55.446	0.067
	F	0.200	1.754	0.007	1.600	13.793	0.080	6.100	46.212	0.179	7.900	69.298	0.094
Luxembourg	M	..	..	..	..	..	..	1.100	9.240	0.034	..	..	..
	F	..	..	..	..	..	..	3.200	23.800	0.100	..	..	..
Netherlands	M	0.900	7.759	0.030	1.600	12.800	0.080	-0.100	-0.709	-0.003	2.400	20.690	0.029
	F	0.700	5.691	0.023	1.700	13.077	0.085	4.300	29.252	0.130	6.700	54.472	0.081
New Zealand	M	0.700	5.738	0.023	0.000	0.000	0.000	0.700	5.426	0.021	1.400	11.475	0.017
	F	0.500	3.759	0.017	1.000	7.246	0.050	2.700	18.243	0.082	4.200	31.579	0.051
Norway	M	0.200	1.481	0.007	1.200	8.759	0.060	-0.400	-2.685	-0.012	1.000	7.407	0.012
	F	0.200	1.389	0.007	1.400	9.589	0.070	2.700	16.875	0.082	4.300	29.861	0.052
Portugal	M	..	..	..	..	..	..	1.800	15.130	0.056	..	..	..
	F	..	..	..	..	..	..	2.800	20.000	0.088	..	..	..
Spain	M	1.400	15.556	0.047	1.600	15.385	0.080	2.400	20.000	0.083	5.400	60.000	0.068
	F	2.300	25.000	0.077	2.500	21.739	0.125	3.500	25.000	0.121	8.300	90.217	0.105
Sweden	M	0.400	3.125	0.013	0.300	2.273	0.015	1.100	8.148	0.034	1.800	14.062	0.022
	F	0.200	1.460	0.007	0.400	2.878	0.020	3.900	27.273	0.122	4.500	32.847	0.055
Switzerland	M	0.900	8.911	0.030	1.400	12.727	0.070	3.100	25.000	0.091	5.400	53.465	0.064
	F	1.400	13.084	0.047	1.900	15.702	0.095	5.800	41.429	0.171	9.100	85.047	0.108
United Kingdom	M	0.500	4.630	0.017	0.700	6.195	0.035	1.100	9.167	0.034	2.300	21.296	0.028
	F	1.100	9.167	0.037	1.300	9.924	0.065	2.800	19.444	0.087	5.200	43.333	0.063
United States	M	0.200	1.739	0.007	1.000	8.547	0.050	1.900	14.961	0.059	3.100	26.957	0.038
	F	0.600	4.918	0.020	2.200	17.187	0.110	4.100	27.333	0.128	6.900	56.557	0.084
Average	M	0.805	7.461	0.027	0.816	7.088	0.041	1.347	11.209	0.042	2.968	27.853	0.036
	F	1.089	9.795	0.036	1.268	10.005	0.063	3.784	26.714	0.117	6.142	53.065	0.075
Range	M	2.500	23.469	0.083	2.400	22.135	0.120	4.900	42.863	0.144	4.600	52.593	0.056
	F	2.900	27.184	0.096	2.600	22.485	0.130	3.600	29.337	0.099	4.900	60.356	0.058
Standard Deviation	M	0.569	5.573	0.019	0.706	6.171	0.035	1.206	10.442	0.036	1.329	14.644	0.016
	F	0.780	7.784	0.026	0.670	5.637	0.034	0.974	7.582	0.028	1.351	12.515	0.016

Source: Table 11.

years, in 1950 by 4.2 years and in the early 1980s by 6.8 years. Similarly, differences in life expectancy at age 40 have increased from 2.1 years in 1900 and 1930, to 3.1 years in 1950 and to 5.6 years in 1980. Life expectancy differences at age 65 have increased from 0.8 year in 1900, to 1.1 in 1930, to 1.6 in 1950 and to 4 years in the early 1980s.

Much of this increase in the female versus male life expectancy can be attributed to greater reductions in female mortality, especially in the higher age ranges. These reductions have widened the gap in life expectancy at birth. It is estimated that 50-60 per cent of the increase in differential life expectancy at birth can be attributed to diverging male-female death rates from cancer and cardiovascular disease[11].

The actual causal factors accounting for differential life expectancy among women and men are both biological and environmental. These include: lifestyles, working conditions and societally-determined sex roles. There is also strong evidence that the higher incidence of cigarette smoking among males is especially important[12].

There are, however, still significant cross-country differences in life expectancy, despite the fact that variations in life expectancy around the OECD average have decreased over time. For males, in 1900 life expectancy at birth ranged from 34 years in Spain to 58 years in New Zealand. By the 1980s the range (excluding Turkey) was from 69 in Portugal and Luxembourg to 75 in Japan. For females, in 1900 life expectancy at birth ranged from 36 in Spain to 61 in New Zealand. By the 1980s life expectancy (excluding Turkey) ranged from 76 in Ireland, Portugal and Luxembourg to 81 in Iceland, Japan and Switzerland. The largest annual increases over the 1900-1980s period took place in Austria, Italy, Japan and Spain.

Similar trends in life expectancy at age 40 and age 65 are observed. In 1900 life expectancy for males at age 40 ranged from 26 years or less in Austria, Japan, Spain and Switzerland to 31 years or more in Ireland and Norway. In 1980, life expectancy for males at age 40 ranged from less than 32 years in Finland and Luxembourg to more than 36 years in Greece and Iceland. For females, in 1900 life expectancy at 40 ranged from 26 years in Spain to 32 years or more in New Zealand, Norway and Sweden. By 1980 the range was from 36 years in Ireland to 41 or more in Canada and Iceland. Austria, Japan, Spain and Switzerland had the largest increases over the 80-year period.

Life expectancy at age 65 for males in 1900 ranged from less than 10 years in Spain to over 12 years in New Zealand, Norway and Sweden. In the early 1980s the range was from less than 13 years in Belgium and Ireland to more than 15 years in Greece, Iceland, Japan and Switzerland. For females life expectancy at age 65 in 1900 varied from 9 years in Spain to 13 or more years in Denmark, Iceland, New Zealand, Norway and Sweden. In the early 1980s the range was from less than 16 years in Ireland to 19 or more years in Iceland, Japan,

the Netherlands, Switzerland and the United States. The countries with the largest increases between 1900-1980s were Japan, Spain and Switzerland.

It is difficult to attribute improvements in life expectancy and reductions in mortality to specific causal factors. Studies in several countries have tended to show that higher standards of living and education are related to reductions in mortality. Medical care has generally been found to be a less important determinant of such reductions[13]. Interestingly, however, at a cross-national level there does appear to be a statistically significant inverse relationship between per capita health spending and infant mortality for the OECD countries. Moreover, per capita health expenditures also are related statistically significantly, and directly, to life expectancies in women but not men.

Charts 4 and 5 display the inverse relationships between per capita health expenditures and infant mortality rates for males and females. Higher expenditures are associated with lower infant mortality rates. The calculated elasticities both for men and for women of -0.6 indicate that a 10 per cent higher per capita health expenditure is associated with a 6 per cent lower infant mortality rate. Differences in per capita health expenditures alone account for 46 per cent of the variation in male and female infant mortality rates. Intuitively, these results are not surprising for several reasons. First, as shown in Chapter 7, countries with higher levels of health expenditures also have higher GDPs, and hence one would expect higher standards of living (nutrition, housing, heating, etc.). Second, countries which spend more on their health systems are likely to have greater availability of specific technologies such as neo-natal intensive care units, which can substantially increase infant survival rates. Third, such countries are also likely to spend more on programmes affecting the health of pregnant women (pre- and post-natal examinations, targeted public health programmes, education programmes, etc.).

Also of interest is the relationship between per capita health expenditures and life expectancies at birth, age 40, and age 65. The simple correlations for males are 0.35, 0.14, and 0.33, respectively. The respective correlations for female life expectancies are 0.60, 0.42, and 0.66. While the correlations for males are relatively small and not statistically significantly different from zero, the correlations for females are larger and statistically significant. This suggests that higher per capita health expenditures are directly associated with longer life expectancies for women but not men. Perhaps this is due to differences in societal roles, which result in life expectancies for men being more closely related to occupational and other social, as opposed to health systems-specific, factors than for women. Perhaps the morbidity patterns of women are more amenable to therapeutic health systems' interventions than those of men. Alternatively, the simple model employed here may be mis-specified with life expectancies being dependent on other social and economic factors that are

Chart 4

MALE INFANT DEATH RATES
VERSUS PER CAPITA HEALTH SPENDING IN PPPs

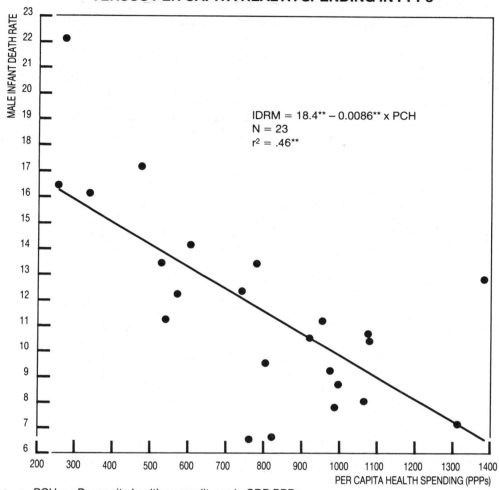

$$IDRM = 18.4^{**} - 0.0086^{**} \times PCH$$
$$N = 23$$
$$r^2 = .46^{**}$$

Notes : PCH = Per capita health expenditures in GDP PPPs.
IDRM = Infant death rates for males.
** = Statistically significant at .05 level.
N = Number of countries.
r^2 = Adjusted correlation coefficient squared.
Excludes Turkey.
Per capita health expenditure figures are for the same years as the respective infant mortality figures.

Sources : Table 8.
Measuring Health Care 1960-1983, OECD, Paris, 1985.
Figures for 1984 are preliminary OECD estimates.

strongly related (or not related) to per capita health spending. Clearly, a simple analysis of the type undertaken here cannot answer these questions. A far more complex model embodying various social, economic and medical factors is needed.

Causes of Death

As discussed above, increased life expectancy has been associated with significant changes in morbidity patterns. Unfortunately, given the well-known difficulties in the measurement and accuracy of morbidity indicators, it is problematic to do detailed statistical comparisons over long-time periods. Thus, for purposes of this analysis, only current differences in morbidity patterns, measured in terms of causes of death, are analysed in detail, while historical changes are discussed in a more general context.

From a historical perspective, the principal causes of death in the developed countries have shifted from acute infectious diseases to chronic diseases. There has been a

Chart 5

FEMALE INFANT DEATH RATES
VERSUS PER CAPITA HEALTH SPENDING IN PPPs

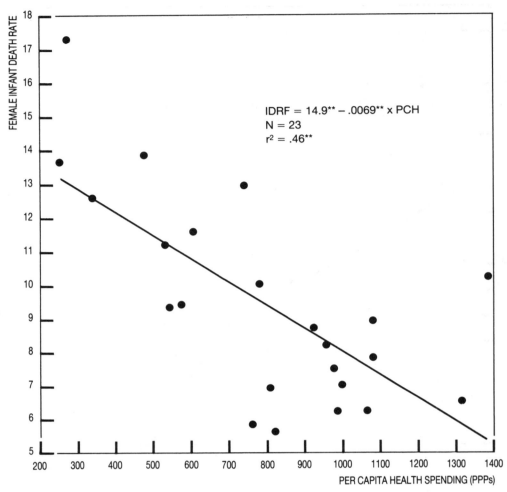

IDRF = 14.9** − .0069** x PCH
N = 23
r^2 = .46**

Notes : Same as Chart 4.
IDRF = Infant death rates for females.

Source : Same as Chart 4.

substantial decline in acute causes of death in OECD countries during this century. While the timing of these declines and current causes of death may differ across OECD countries, the overall trends and causes are similar. One study of 12 OECD countries found reductions in mortality rates from infectious, parasitic, and respiratory diseases of between 56 to 81 per cent from the mid-1930s to the mid-1950s[14]. Today, these diseases are only of minor significance for all age groups, except the elderly, for whom influenza and pneumonia are still significant causes of death.

The four major causes of death in Europe are diseases of the circulatory system, cancer, external causes, and diseases of the respiratory system. In particular, the dominant lethal conditions are heart disease, malignant neoplasms, cerebrovascular disease, influenza and pneumonia, arteriosclerosis, diabetes, bronchitis, and emphysema. Severe chronic conditions such as hypertension, mental illness and depression, arthritis, other conditions of the musculoskeletal system, sensory impairments, and edentulism are often non-lethal, but contribute to functional disability or, in the case of hypertension, to death from the above mentioned causes[15].

While cardiovascular disease mortality has decreased overall, it has generally increased for males between 1960 and 1970 and remained unchanged since then.

Deaths due to ischemic heart disease have been decreasing overall, but increasing in males under 65. Deaths from cerebrovascular disease have been declining. Cancer mortality is generally increasing largely due to increased mortality from lung cancer, although mortality from most other cancers (e.g. cervix) are declining. Deaths from external causes (e.g. accidents, suicides, homicides, poisonings) have been declining, although there has been some increase in deaths from suicides[16].

Table 15 contains age-adjusted death rates (using the European age structure) for 23 OECD countries (excluding Turkey) for the following causes of death: Infectious and Parasitic Diseases, Malignant Neoplasms, Diseases of the Circulatory System, Diseases of the Respiratory System, Diseases of the Digestive System, Injury and Poisoning, and All Causes.

These data should not be interpreted too precisely for several reasons. First, they apply to different years (1980 to 1984) for different countries. Second, the data on specific causes are subject to small yearly fluctuations (e.g. an influenza epidemic). Third, the categories presented are highly aggregated. For example, the category Injury and Poisoning includes accidents of all kinds, homicides, suicides, etc. Fourth, death often results from multiple causes, only one of which is reported, and reporting can be biased by cultural factors. Nevertheless, these data can be analysed to obtain a general indication of differences in causes of death across OECD countries.

The age-standardised OECD average death rate (deaths per 100 000 population) is 855, ranging from a low of 699 in Japan to a high of 1 054 in Ireland. The coefficient of variation of 0.11 indicates a relatively small dispersion of death rates around the average. For men, the average death rate is 1 114, varying from a low of 899 in Japan to a high of 1359 in Luxembourg. The coefficient of variation of 0.11 indicates about the same dispersion around the mean in the death rates for men as in the overall population and for women, where the rates averaged 663 and ranged from a low of 542 in Switzerland to a high of 843 in Ireland with a coefficient of variation of 0.12.

With respect to causes of death, Diseases of the Circulatory System and Malignant Neoplasms are the first and second most important causes of death in every OECD country accounting on average for 46 and 23 per cent of all deaths, respectively. Injury and Poisoning (12 countries) and Diseases of the Respiratory System (11 countries) are the third major causes of death. Deaths from Infectious and Parasitic Diseases are of minor importance.

The distributions for All Causes of Death, Malignant Neoplasms, and Diseases of the Circulatory System (coefficients of variation of 0.11, 0.13, and 0.16) are rather condensed, while deaths from Infectious and Parasitic Diseases (0.40), Diseases of the Respiratory System (0.39), Diseases of the Digestive System (0.36) and Injury and Poisoning (0.23) display much more variability across countries. The same trends are found for cause-specific death rates for males and females.

Concerning the two leading causes of death, Portugal, Greece and Spain have the lowest overall death rates from Malignant Neoplasms, while Greece, Spain and Japan have the lowest female death rates. Belgium, Denmark and Luxembourg have the highest overall rates, and Denmark, Ireland and New Zealand have the highest female death rates. For males, Portugal, Sweden and Greece have the lowest death rates and Belgium, Luxembourg and the Netherlands the highest. For Diseases of the Circulatory System, France, Japan and Switzerland have the lowest overall death rates; France, Iceland and Japan have the lowest female death rates; and France, Japan and Greece have the lowest male death rates. Ireland, Austria and Finland have the highest overall and male death rates, while Ireland, Austria and Luxembourg have the highest female death rates.

To rather simplistically analyse the relation between causes of death and expenditures on health, Charts 6 to 8 display overall death rates for All Causes, Malignant Neoplasms, and Diseases of the Circulatory System against per capita health spending. The relationships are quite weak. Only in the case of death rates for All Causes is the relationship statistically significant, and even in this case variations in per capita health expenditures account for only 21 per cent of the variation in death rates for All Causes. The relationship is negative, higher per capita health expenditures are associated with lower death rates. There are no statistically significant relationships between death rates from Malignant Neoplasms or Diseases of the Circulatory System and per capita health expenditures.

Table 16 contains the elasticities of death rates (for all seven causes for total population, males and females) relative to per capita health expenditures. The elasticities are quite small, exceeding 0.3 (in absolute value terms) in only 3 of the 21 cases and never exceeding 0.4. In fact, in only 5 of the 21 cases are the elasticities statistically significantly different from 0. For 5 of the seven causes of death, the elasticities are negative indicating higher per capita health expenditures are (weakly if at all) related to lower death rates. The positive relationships found for Malignant Neoplasms and Injury and Poisoning may be indicative of the importance of other societal factors (smoking, stress, urbanisation, etc.) in influencing death rates from these causes. Nevertheless, overall the relationships are extremely weak. Both from perspectives of statistical significance and the magnitude of the elasticities, there does not appear to be much relationship between aggregate death rates and per capita health spending.

The low elasticities and lack of statistically significant relationships are not surprising. As discussed above, given the numerous economic, medical, social and historical factors that affect health, as well as the aggregate nature of the cause of death categories, a far more sophisticated model and a far more detailed

Table 15

AGE-STANDARDISED DEATH RATES PER 100 000

Country	Year	Sex	Infectious & Parasitic Diseases (01-07)	Malignant Neoplasm (08-14)	Diseases of the Circulatory System (25-30)	Diseases of the Respiratory System (31-32)	Diseases of the Digestive System (33-34)	Injury & Poisoning (E47-E56)	All Causes
Australia	1983	T	4.2	191.5	414.0	58.4	27.9	50.5	820.8
		M	5.5	249.8	526.0	96.4	36.8	73.6	1 073.5
		F	3.3	150.7	323.6	35.1	20.7	28.5	628.3
Austria	1984	T	4.5	209.3	468.5	43.6	54.3	80.6	934.4
		M	7.3	276.3	593.1	69.1	80.7	120.9	1 229.9
		F	2.5	171.0	387.1	30.1	34.4	44.6	736.3
Belgium	1984	T	6.4	229.7	375.4	64.0	35.8	68.2	918.9
		M	8.3	323.0	481.6	112.0	44.0	91.3	1 214.5
		F	5.0	166.2	298.4	33.4	29.0	46.3	705.0
Canada	1984	T	4.3	199.1	339.6	55.3	29.4	56.0	761.8
		M	5.2	254.2	445.4	86.7	37.2	81.9	1 002.5
		F	3.7	159.3	255.7	34.9	22.9	31.7	575.9
Denmark	1984	T	3.2	234.3	388.0	62.0	28.7	69.3	884.2
		M	3.8	281.1	510.9	88.4	36.0	87.3	1 127.0
		F	2.6	203.4	293.5	44.7	22.2	51.8	699.6
Finland	1983	T	7.9	186.7	476.5	69.1	23.7	75.7	912.9
		M	11.2	264.2	654.8	117.4	31.0	121.5	1 277.3
		F	6.1	144.1	356.1	44.0	17.9	36.7	674.2
France	1983	T	10.5	205.5	274.7	51.5	54.0	83.4	825.4
		M	14.3	300.6	355.8	80.1	74.5	116.4	1 121.0
		F	7.9	136.4	215.3	34.5	37.5	52.4	604.0
Germany	1984	T	6.0	205.2	423.0	52.1	43.7	55.1	877.4
		M	8.4	274.0	556.5	87.9	60.6	75.8	1 172.1
		F	4.5	166.5	339.3	33.7	31.3	36.0	691.2
Greece	1983	T	7.4	160.5	366.2	52.6	30.3	48.7	817.6
		M	9.7	217.0	402.9	66.1	39.8	68.3	962.1
		F	5.6	114.5	332.2	41.9	22.3	29.9	692.2
Iceland	1983	T	4.1	188.1	360.6	66.6	16.1	64.1	750.4
		M	4.2	222.1	505.1	80.2	15.6	95.4	977.3
		F	4.4	162.7	231.6	56.0	16.8	33.1	552.4
Ireland	1982	T	8.3	209.7	536.6	136.9	27.3	50.7	1 054.4
		M	11.5	247.2	674.8	180.3	31.3	72.0	1 312.4
		F	5.5	181.6	420.8	105.2	24.2	29.5	843.3
Italy	1981	T	5.2	197.7	401.7	62.7	52.5	48.7	869.5
		M	7.3	269.3	490.5	96.4	76.9	70.0	1 123.3
		F	3.6	143.6	333.8	40.3	32.8	28.7	675.0
Japan	1984	T	10.7	164.7	285.7	62.5	35.3	49.7	699.4
		M	15.5	226.2	344.9	92.7	48.1	73.0	898.7
		F	7.2	120.0	242.2	43.0	24.6	28.5	550.2
Luxembourg	1982	T	5.0	256.6	467.6	41.8	55.0	86.1	1 028.4
		M	6.5	372.8	590.0	63.9	64.1	124.4	1 358.7
		F	3.7	179.8	380.2	28.1	46.3	53.4	793.7
Netherlands	1984	T	4.2	220.9	341.2	53.2	27.6	40.4	784.5
		M	5.2	308.0	457.0	86.3	32.7	52.9	1 054.7
		F	3.5	160.9	254.5	32.8	23.5	28.7	588.2
New Zealand	1983	T	4.9	213.7	442.3	104.3	23.9	52.8	922.5
		M	5.7	260.7	577.4	150.8	29.3	73.0	1 185.6
		F	4.2	181.9	338.8	74.9	19.7	32.8	726.8
Norway	1984	T	5.1	178.2	368.2	64.8	22.6	54.4	785.4
		M	6.3	223.3	496.4	86.6	27.4	97.5	1 030.8
		F	4.0	147.4	264.4	49.8	18.9	31.8	592.2
Portugal	1984	T	10.2	154.0	422.0	68.4	50.2	73.2	978.0
		M	15.3	202.4	506.1	101.3	76.9	114.2	1 249.5
		F	6.1	120.8	360.2	46.2	29.1	36.6	773.3
Spain	1980	T	10.9	162.6	378.1	76.2	49.4	43.0	820.5
		M	14.7	221.6	445.1	109.7	70.6	64.6	1 038.7
		F	7.9	119.6	325.8	53.5	32.3	22.9	653.2

Table 15 (Cont'd)

AGE-STANDARDISED DEATH RATES PER 100 000

Country	Year	Sex	Infectious & Parasitic Diseases (01-07)	Malignant Neoplasm (08-14)	Diseases of the Circulatory System (25-30)	Diseases of the Respiratory System (31-32)	Diseases of the Digestive System (33-34)	Injury & Poisoning (E47-E56)	All Causes
Sweden	1984	T	4.8	168.5	394.3	50.2	21.7	54.2	757.5
		M	5.9	202.2	517.7	69.3	28.0	77.9	977.7
		F	4.0	145.8	295.4	37.5	16.3	31.5	583.0
Switzerland	1984	T	4.7	194.9	314.3	33.5	25.7	68.0	711.7
		M	5.8	260.9	406.3	54.1	34.9	95.8	938.4
		F	4.0	149.7	245.7	20.1	18.0	42.0	541.8
United Kingdom*	1983	T	3.6	217.6	435.2	130.5	25.1	35.0	915.8
		M	4.5	279.1	569.6	185.2	28.0	46.5	1 189.3
		F	2.9	179.6	333.1	100.0	22.8	23.7	725.9
United States	1982	T	8.4	193.3	407.0	53.2	32.7	62.2	842.4
		M	10.4	247.1	531.4	81.4	41.7	95.1	1 107.0
		F	7.0	156.9	314.0	35.3	25.2	32.3	645.7
Mean		T	6.3	197.5	394.8	65.8	34.5	59.6	855.4
Range			7.7	102.6	261.9	103.4	38.9	51.1	355.0
Standard Deviation			2.5	25.7	62.4	25.5	12.3	14.0	94.6
Mean		M	8.4	260.1	506.1	97.5	45.5	86.5	1 114.0
Range			11.7	170.6	329.9	131.1	65.1	77.9	460.0
Standard Deviation			3.7	40.7	84.7	33.8	19.5	22.0	126.1
Mean		F	4.7	154.9	310.5	45.9	25.6	35.4	663.1
Range			5.4	88.9	205.5	85.1	30.0	30.5	301.5
Standard Deviation			1.6	23.1	54.0	21.1	7.5	8.9	82.4

Notes: * England and Wales. Numbers in parentheses refer to ICD-9 disease codes. Death rates are standardised on the basis of a European Standardised population. T - total population. M - males. F - females.

Source: World Health Statistics, 1983, 1984, 1985, World Health Organisation, Geneva, 1983, 1984, 1985. Updated statistics for several countries were provided by the World Health Organisation to the OECD Secretariat.

analysis that goes well beyond the scope of this report would be needed to systematically and scientifically explore these relationships. Nevertheless, societal morbidity patterns do impose significant economic costs on both health and economic systems.

Table 16

ELASTICITY OF DEATH RATES
TO PER CAPITA HEALTH EXPENDITURES

Cause of Death	All Individuals	Males	Females
Infectious and Parasitic Diseases	-0.320 (0.11)	-0.399 (0.14)*	-0.178 (0.01)
Malignant Neoplasms	0.103 (0.09)	0.086 (0.02)	0.140 (0.13)*
Diseases of the Circulatory System	-0.097 (0.03)	-0.009 (-0.05)	-0.198 (0.22)*
Diseases of the Respiratory System	-0.275 (0.10)	-0.214 (0.06)	-0.328 (0.11)
Diseases of the Digestive System	-0.234 (0.05)	-0.299 (0.06)	-0.136 (0.01)
Injury and Poisoning	0.096 (-0.01)	0.091 (-0.02)	0.129 (0.02)
All Causes	-0.103 (0.14)*	-0.057 (0.01)	-0.153 (0.28)*

Notes: Calculated by regressing the logarithms of per capita health expenditures denominated in US$ on the basis of GDP PPPs on the logarithms of death rates.
* = Statistically significant at a 0.05 or higher level.
( ) = Adjusted correlation coefficient squared.

Sources: Same as Chart 6.

Costs of Illness

In evaluating the economic burden of illness both direct and indirect, as well as present and future, costs should be analysed. Direct costs of illness are defined as the health and non-health (e.g. meals, transportation) care direct costs incurred to prevent, diagnose and treat illnesses, and to restore function. Indirect costs are the value of production lost and increased non-market household costs (e.g. spouses' assistance at home) due to morbidity, disability and premature death. In principle, direct costs should also include some valuation for pain and suffering, and lost production costs should be adjusted for productivity changes. Due to valuation problems, these factors are rarely included.

A distinction is also made between studies which focus on disease prevalence – the cost consequences of all illness during the year independent of its initial onset, and studies which focus on disease incidence – the current and future cost consequences of illness which occur for the first time in the base year. Incidence studies are more difficult from data perspectives, because they require information on the future medical cost consequences of the onset of specific diseases in the base year. Such studies are useful for evaluating the benefits derived from preventing a specific disease. The most common approach, and the one employed in all the studies below, is the prevalence approach. All studies

Chart 6

DEATH RATES (ALL CAUSES)
VERSUS PER CAPITA HEALTH SPENDING IN PPPs

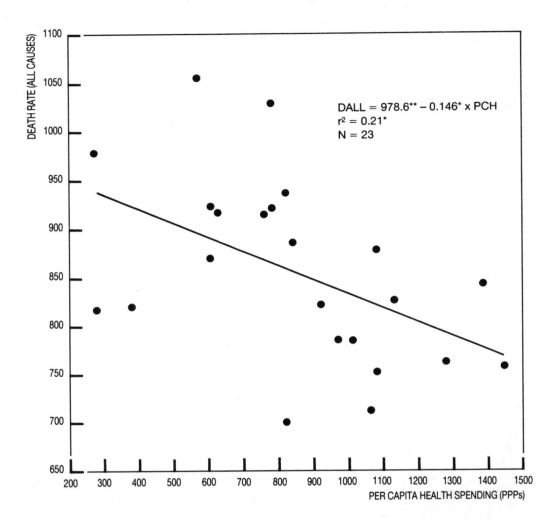

Notes : PCH = Per capita health expenditures in GDP PPPs.
DALL = Overall death rates for All Causes.
N = Number of observations.
** = Statistically significant at .01 level.
* = Statistically significant at .05 level.
r^2 = Adjusted correlation coefficient squared.
Per capita expenditures are for the same years as the death rates.
Excludes Turkey.

Sources : Table 15.
Measuring Health Care 1960-1983, OECD, Paris, 1985, and OECD Secretariat estimates for 1984.

also assume full employment and generally assume equality of marginal and average wage rates, assumptions of questionable validity in times of protracted economic recession.

In practice most studies for a variety of methodological, data, and valuation reasons, employ the prevalence approach, concentrate on direct medical costs only, and do not account for pain and suffering. Moreover, the results are often sensitive to the interest rate chosen for discounting future lost production costs and non-market household production. In the simplest cases the direct medical care costs, as presented in national health

Chart 7

DEATH RATES DUE TO MALIGNANT NEOPLASMS
VERSUS PER CAPITA HEALTH SPENDING IN PPPs

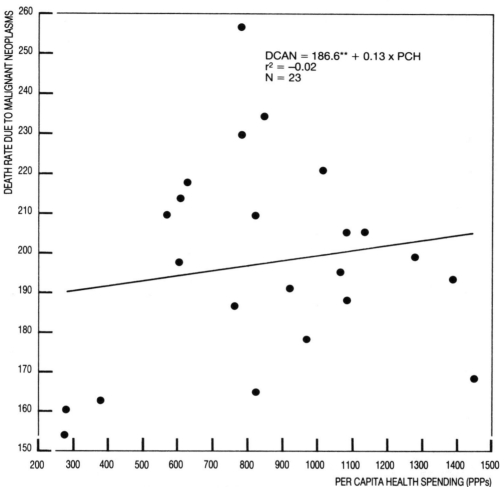

$$DCAN = 186.6^{**} + 0.13 \times PCH$$
$$r^2 = -0.02$$
$$N = 23$$

Notes : DCAN = Overall death rate for Malignant Neoplasms.
Same as Chart 6.

Source : Same as Chart 6.

accounts, are partitioned by disease categories, other demographic factors and, sometimes, by type of service and source of payment. One should, however, interpret the results below with caution given the differences in base years and discount rates as well as differences in methodologies (cost proportioning algorithms, valuation of household production, etc.). More generally, differences in costs by disease categories can result from these methodological differences as well as differences in disease prevalence, demography, medical practice patterns, medical care supply factors, wage levels, price levels and relatives, etc.

Data for cost of illness by disease category are presented for Finland (1972), Germany (1980), Sweden (1975), the United States (1980) and Japan (1977, 1980, 1983)[17]. The studies for Finland, Germany, Sweden and the United States employ generally similar methodologies in terms of calculating both the direct medical care costs in the base year and the indirect base year and future lost production costs due to mortality and morbidity. The direct costs for Finland include only hospital costs, which account for about 44 per cent of total direct costs, and indirect costs are not discounted. The discount rate presented here for calculating indirect costs for Sweden, Germany and the United States is 4 per cent. The indirect costs in the

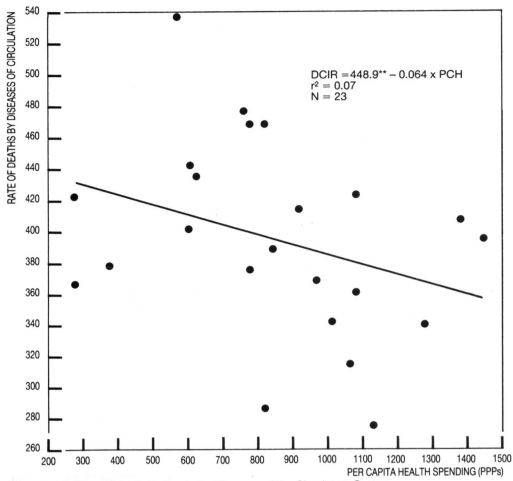

Chart 8

**DEATH RATES DUE TO DISEASES OF THE CIRCULATORY SYSTEM
VERSUS PER CAPITA HEALTH SPENDING IN PPPs**

DCIR = 448.9** − 0.064 x PCH
r² = 0.07
N = 23

Notes : DCIR = Overall death rate for Diseases of the Circulatory System.
Same as Chart 6.

Source : Same as Chart 6.

German study do not include non-market household production costs. The Japanese study provides information on the direct costs only, disaggregated by type of service and demographic factors.

Table 17 contains the percentages of total, direct and indirect costs allocated by the main 18 ICD disease categories. Direct costs represent medical care costs allocated to each disease category. Despite differences in the rank ordering of direct costs among individual disease categories, there are similarities in terms of the most costly illnesses. Diseases of the Circulatory System was the highest cost category in the United States and Japan, and the second highest in Finland, Germany and Sweden. Mental Disorders was the highest direct cost category in Sweden and Finland, third in the United States, and sixth in Japan and Germany. Diseases of the Digestive System was the second highest cost category in the United States, Japan and Sweden (along with Diseases of the Circulatory System), first in Germany, and sixth in Finland. Accidents, Poisoning and Violence was also a significantly high cost category, fourth in the United States and Sweden, fifth in Finland, third in Germany and eighth in Japan.

Indirect costs are heavily influenced by the incidence of disease by age and sex, wage rates, the discount rate, valuation of non-market costs, etc. The relationship

Table 17

COSTS OF ILLNESS IN FIVE OECD COUNTRIES
(Percentage of costs allocated by disease category)

	Finland (72)			Sweden (75)			United States (80)			Japan			Germany (80)		
	T	D	I	T	D	I	T	D	I	D(77)	D(80)	D(83)	T	D	I
1. Infective and parasitic diseases	3.0	7.6	2.4	2.0	1.5	2.2	2.3	2.0	2.4	4.8	3.5	3.2	2.7	3.0	2.4
2. Neoplasms	5.3	6.9	5.1	7.4	5.3	8.3	11.1	6.2	15.4	6.2	7.9	8.9	7.0	4.4	10.1
3. Endocrine and metabolic diseases	1.7	2.4	1.6	2.2	2.5	2.1	2.8	3.5	2.3	2.8	3.1	3.5	2.6	3.6	1.4
4. Diseases of the blood	0.2	0.7	0.1	0.3	0.4	0.3	0.5	0.5	0.4	0.6	0.7	0.9	0.3	0.2	0.4
5. Mental disorders	17.8	23.3	17.1	14.6	15.7	14.2	6.7	9.4	4.5	7.6	7.1	7.1	4.4	5.1	3.7
6. Diseases of the nervous system	4.2	4.1	4.2	4.1	4.4	4.0	5.1	8.1	2.4	6.6	5.5	5.8	4.2	4.8	3.5
7. Diseases of the circulatory system	24.2	17.1	25.0	15.3	13.7	16.0	18.7	15.4	21.5	19.7	21.2	22.8	15.2	15.0	15.4
8. Diseases of the respiratory system	4.7	5.3	4.6	7.9	5.1	9.1	7.3	7.9	6.8	10.6	10.6	8.9	8.0	5.6	10.8
9. Diseases of the digestive system	2.2	6.3	1.7	7.9	13.7	5.3	9.3	14.7	4.7	14.2	13.1	13.0	19.9	28.6	9.7
10. Diseases of the genito-urinary system	1.1	4.1	0.8	2.5	3.6	1.9	3.4	5.8	1.3	6.9	8.4	6.6	3.4	4.2	2.4
11. Complications of pregnancy and childbirth	0.7	5.9	0.2	1.0	2.6	0.4				1.4	1.2	1.2	2.2	3.3	0.8
12. Diseases of the skin and subcutaneous tissue	0.4	1.0	0.4	1.0	1.5	0.8	1.5	2.8	0.3	3.0	2.2	2.1	1.6	1.9	1.3
13. Diseases of the musculoskeletal system and connective tissue	16.4	4.8	17.7	15.1	5.3	19.4	4.5	6.2	3.1	6.3	7.1	7.2	9.5	7.6	11.7
14. Congenital anomalies	2.1	1.0	2.2	0.8	0.4	1.0	1.4	0.6	2.0	0.5	0.5	0.4	0.6	0.3	1.0
15. Certain causes of perinatal morbidity and mortality	1.8	0.5	2.0	0.5	0.3	0.5				0.2	0.2	0.3	0.6	0.3	1.0
16. Symptoms and ill-defined conditions	0.5	2.5	0.3	2.2	3.0	1.8	4.3	1.8*	2.8	1.1	0.6	0.8	3.2	2.8	3.6
17. Accidents, poisonings and violence	13.4	6.5	14.2	11.1	7.8	12.7	18.2	8.8	26.4	7.5	7.0	7.2	13.7	7.7	20.7
18. All others and unallocated	0.3	-	0.4	4.1	13.2	-	2.9	6.1	3.8	-	-	-	0.9	1.5	0.1
Total (100%)		(100%)			(100%)			(100%)			(100%)			(100%)	

Notes: T = Total Costs;   D = Direct Costs;   I = Indirect Costs.
*   Includes categories 11 and 15.
( ) Year.

Sources: B. Lindgren, "Les Coûts de la Maladie: Méthode et Résultats", Revue Française de Finances Publiques, No. 2, 1983.
K. Heinke, "Direct and Indirect Cost of Illness, Federal Republic of Germany, 1980", Paper presented at the 11th Colloquium on Health Economics of the Robert Bosch Foundation, Murrhardt, November 1983.
D. Rice, T. Hodgson & A. Kopstein, "The Economic Costs of Illness: A Replication and Update", Health Care Financing Review, Fall 1985.
Japanese Ministry of Health and Welfare, Statistics and Information Department, National Medical Care Expenditure, Tokyo, 1985, pp. 42-43.

between direct and indirect costs as well as the percentage distribution of indirect costs by disease category are of interest. Data not displayed here, but contained in the studies cited, indicate that the indirect costs either approximately equal or exceed the direct costs in all cases. While more precise comparisons of the absolute magnitudes are difficult due to methodological differences, the percentage distributions of indirect costs by disease category are less susceptible to bias from some of these problems.

Since the distribution of indirect costs by disease category is heavily influenced by the age and sex structure of mortality and morbidity, diseases that strike significant numbers of young people resulting in premature death or long-term disability, will result in substantial indirect costs, as opposed to those that affect the retired elderly. Thus the category Accidents, Poisoning and Violence, which is the principal cause of death in young people, has indirect costs that are two to four times the direct medical costs in all four countries with indirect cost data. Cardiovascular problems, one of the principal causes of death in men in the 44-64 age range, which are included under Diseases of the Circulatory System, also display indirect costs substantially in excess of the direct costs in all four countries.

Total costs combine the effects of direct and indirect costs. Total costs for Diseases of the Circulatory System were the highest cost category in Finland, Sweden and the United States, and the second highest in Germany. Diseases of the Digestive System were the highest cost disease category in Germany, the fourth highest in the United States, fifth highest in Sweden and ninth highest in Finland. Accidents, Poisoning and Violence were the fourth highest in Finland and Sweden, second in the United States and third in Germany. Mental Disorders were the second highest in Finland, third in Sweden, sixth in the United States and seventh in Germany. Neoplasms, the second largest cause of death in OECD countries, were the fifth most costly disease in Finland, seventh in Sweden, third in the United States and sixth in Germany.

While it is difficult to make precise statements about these data due to their aggregate nature, some general observations can be made. First, in evaluating health care expenditure policies, the direct as well as indirect costs should be analysed. Basing policy decisions on benefit and coverage changes, implementation of new technologies, and medical research solely on direct cost criteria could lead to substantial misallocations of resources. For example, strictly from a narrow cost perspective, it would appear that the overriding emphasis on cancer and cancer research may be overstated. From total, direct and indirect cost perspectives, cancer is not in the top three disease categories in any of the countries, except for the United States, where it is third for total and indirect costs. Cancer accounts for

5.3 per cent of total costs in Finland, 7.4 in Sweden, 11.1 in the United States and 7.0 in Germany.

Diseases of the Circulatory System are the most costly in terms of total costs for three of the four countries and account for between 15.2 to 24.2 of all illness costs. Policies designed to prevent or treat circulatory diseases such as ischemic heart disease could have significant benefits in terms of productivity gains and reduced medical care resource use. Such policies should undoubtedly contain major components focusing on lifestyles (eating habits, exercise) as well as environment.

Much the same argument can be made about Accidents, Poisoning and Violence which account for between 11.1 to 18.2 per cent of total costs. The high indirect relative to direct cost aspect underlies the prevalence of these problems among the young. As discussed above, suicides have been on the increase in the younger age groups. Policies aimed at education, counselling, seat belt laws, maximum speed limits, laws increasing the drinking age, gun control and increased economic opportunity for the poor and under-privileged, rather than therapeutic or diagnostic medical interventions, would have the greatest benefit potential.

It is difficult to explain some of the significant differences in costs of illness across countries. For example, the total, direct and indirect costs of Mental Illness are substantially higher in Finland and Sweden than in the United States, Japan and Germany. While some of this may be due to study methodology, it may also reflect higher institutionalisation rates, or the use of large expensive mental hospitals instead of less costly smaller institutional or ambulatory treatment settings for mental illness. In a similar vein, it is difficult to explain the relative costliness of digestive diseases in Germany. Perhaps it relates to differences in diet, or as the study author suggests, the relatively high costs of dental care in Germany.

It is also interesting to assess the changes in costs of illness over time. The direct cost data for Japan do not indicate drastic changes in the rank ordering of the costs of various diseases. However, Rice *et al.*[18] in a comparison of trends in costs of illness in the United States in 1963, 1972 and 1980 found some significant changes. Costs of Diseases of the Circulatory System declined progressively over the 1963-80 time period reflecting a decline in death rates. However, the economic costs of Accidents, Poisoning and Violence have risen concomitantly with increased deaths, largely among the young, from these causes, and the economic costs of Neoplasms have also risen along with increased cancer mortality. The authors point out that over this 17-year period total costs of illness rose 350 per cent, direct costs rose 837 per cent (as a result of very high medical care inflation), and indirect costs rose only at 189 per cent, reflecting slower wage relative to medical care cost growth. This has resulted in direct costs becoming an increasingly larger share of total costs. In fact, Rice *et al.* point out that in the United States indirect costs have declined from 8 times those of direct costs in 1900, to 7 times in 1930, to 3 times in 1963, to 1½ times in 1972 and to approximate equality in 1980. In the chapter that follows, the aggregate health expenditure levels and increases resulting from these illness patterns are analysed in the context of economic, demographic and medical sector specific features.

NOTES AND REFERENCES

1. See Walsh McDermott, "Absence of Indicators of the Influence of Its Physicians on a Society's Health", *The American Journal of Medicine*, Vol. 70, April 1981; and Ernest Schroeder, "Concepts of Health and Illness", in A.J. Culyer (ed.), *Health Indicators*, Martin Robertson, Oxford, 1983.

2. Walsh McDermott, "Absence of Indicators of the Influence of Its Physicians on a Society's Health", *Ibid*.

3. Ernest Schroeder, "Concepts of Health and Illness", *op.cit.*

4. See Sidney Katz *et al.*, "Active Life Expectancy", *The New England Journal of Medicine*, Vol. 309, No. 20, Nov. 17, 1983; and Jean-Pierre Poullier, "The Cathedrals of the 21st Century", in *The Future of Health and Health Systems in Industrialised Countries*, Praeger, New York, 1987.

5. J.W. Hurst, "The Scope for Developing Operational Measures of Health Outcome in the Next 5-10 Years", U.K. Department of Health and Social Security, London, 1985; A.J. Culyer (ed.), *Health Indicators*, *op.cit.*; Ethel Shanas and George L. Maddox, "Health, Health Resources, and the Utilisation of Care" in Robert H. Binstock and Ethel Shanas (eds.), *Handbook of Ageing and Social Sciences*, 2nd Edition, Van Nostrand Reinhold Company, Inc, New York, 1985; and Rachel Rosser, "Issues of Measurement in the Design of Health Indicators: A Review", in Binstock and Shanas (eds.), *Ibid*.

6. See J.W. Hurst, "The Scope for Developing Measures of Health Outcome in the Next 5-10 Years", *Ibid*.

7. Robert H. Brook *et al.*, *The Effect of Coinsurance on the Health of Adults*, Rand Corporation, Santa Monica, California, December 1984.

8. See Walsh McDermott, "Absence of Indicators of the Influences of its Physicians on a Society's Health", *op.cit.*; and Jacob S. Siegel and Sally L. Hoover, "Demographic Aspects of the Health of the Elderly to the Year 2000 and Beyond", *World Health Statistics Quarterly*, Vol. 35, Nos. 3,4, 1982.

9. James F. Fries, "Aging, Natural Death, and the Compression of Morbidity", *The New England Journal of Medicine*, Vol. 303, No. 3, July 17, 1980; Jerome J. Avorn, "Medicine, Health and the Geriatric Transformation", *Daedalus*, Vol. 115, Winter 1986; and Sidney Katz *et al.*, "Active Life Expectancy", *op.cit.*

10. See M. Skeet, *Protecting the Health of the Elderly*, Public Health in Europe 18, World Health Organisation, Regional Office for Europe, Copenhagen, 1983.

11. See Alan D. Lopez and Kyo Hanada, "Mortality Patterns and Trends Among the Elderly in Developed Countries", *World Health Statistics*, Vol. 35, Nos. 3/4, 1982.

12. See Jacob S. Siegel and Sally L. Hoover, "Demographic Aspects of the Health of the Elderly to the Year 2000 and Beyond", *op.cit.*

13. There is, however, some evidence to the contrary. See J.W. Hurst, "The Scope for Developing Operational Measures of Health Outcome in the Next 5-10 Years", *op.cit.*; J.W. Hurst, *Financing Health Services in the United States, Canada, and Britain*, King Edward's Hospital Fund, London, 1985; David A. Crozier, "Health Status and Medical Care Utilisation", *Health Affairs*, Spring 1985; and Steven H. Chapman, Mitchell P. Laplante and Gail Wilensky, "Life Expectancy and Health Status of the Aged", *Social Security Bulletin*, Vol. 49, No. 10, October 1986.

14. See Donald J. Bogue, *Principles of Demography*, John Wiley and Sons Inc., New York, 1969, pp. 580-81.

15. Jacob S. Siegel and Sally L. Hoover, "Demographic Aspects of the Health of the Elderly to the Year 2000 and Beyond", *op.cit.*

16. *Seventh Report on the World Health Situation - Volume 5*, World Health Organisation, Regional Office for Europe, Copenhagen, 1986.

17. See B. Lindgren, "Les Coûts de la Maladie: Méthodes et Résultats", *Revue Française de Finances Publiques*, No. 2, 1983; K. Heinke, "Direct and Indirect Cost of Illness, Federal Republic of Germany, 1980", Paper presented at the 11th Colloquium on Health Economics of the Robert Bosch Foundation, Murrhardt, November 1983; D. Rice, T. Hodgson and A. Kopstein, "The Economic Costs of Illness: A Replication and Update", *Health Care Financing Review,* Fall 1985; and Japanese Ministry of Health and Welfare, Statistics and Information Department, *National Medical Care Expenditure*, Tokyo, 1983.

18. D. Rice, T. Hodgson, and A. Kopstein, "The Economic Costs of Illness: A Replication and Update", *Ibid.*

Chapter 5

SIZE AND GROWTH OF THE HEALTH SECTOR

This chapter analyses the size of and changes in public and overall health expenditures in OECD countries. First, the ratios of total health expenditures to GDP and public health expenditures to total health expenditures are analysed. Second, differences in absolute levels of health expenditures are discussed. Third, changes in real health expenditures relative to changes in real GDP are analysed. Fourth, changes in nominal health expenditures are decomposed into changes in prices, population, and utilisation and intensity of services.

Share of Health in GDP and the Public Share

Table 18 contains data on the ratio of total health expenditures to GDP, as well as the ratio of public to total health spending. Health spending for the OECD (18 countries) has increased from 4.2 per cent of GDP in 1960, to 5.8 per cent in 1970, to 7.0 per cent in 1975, to 7.2 per cent in 1980 and 7.5 per cent in 1984. Interestingly, the health share in GDP appears to have remained constant between 1982 and 1984 at 7.5 per cent. For the major seven OECD countries, the share of health in GDP has increased from 4.4 per cent in 1960, to 5.8 in 1970, to 7.0 in 1975, to 7.4 in 1980 and to 8.0 in 1982 and 1984. Much of this growth took place in the 1960s and early 1970s as public systems and private health insurance expanded in a climate of general economic prosperity. Growth slowed in the late 1970s after the oil shocks, mainly because most public systems had reached maturity, and slow economic growth limited the ability of governments to finance new health expenditures. Indeed, the growth in the GDP share of health has been slower in the 1980s than in any other period. Furthermore, saturation in terms of public coverage has virtually been reached since, as shown in Table 19, public coverage ratios for hospital care increased from an OECD average of 75.3 in 1960 to 88.3 in 1970 to 93.5 in 1975 to 95.1 in 1980 and to 95.3 in 1983.

Nevertheless, there are still significant differences in GDP shares across countries and in the change in shares over time. In 1984, the United States (10.7), Sweden (9.4), and France (9.1) had the highest GDP shares, while Greece (4.6), Portugal (5.5), and New Zealand (5.6), had the lowest. Furthermore, while all countries experienced significant growth in shares between the 1960s and the early 1980s, the rates of growth and their timing differed. By the mid-1980s France, Ireland, Japan, the Netherlands, Spain, Sweden, Switzerland and the United States had experienced at least a doubling of their health expenditures to GDP ratios. On the other hand, Australia, Canada, Greece, Iceland and the United Kingdom had experienced increases of less than 60 per cent.

Public expenditures as a percent of total health spending also increased from an OECD average of 61 per cent in 1960 to 79 per cent in 1984. Most of the growth in the public share had occurred by 1975, when the public share reached 76 per cent. Between 1975 and 1980 the public share increased by only 3 percentage points and has remained virtually unchanged since then. This is consistent with expansion of public programmes in the 1960s and saturation in the late 1970s. One current policy question is whether this levelling-off in the public share will be followed by a decline, as individual countries seek to cope with their health care financing problems by restricting public expenditures and relying on private financing.

Public shares vary widely among countries from a low of 41 per cent in the United States to 80 per cent or more in Australia, Belgium, Denmark, Iceland, Ireland, Italy, Norway, Sweden and the United Kingdom. Growth in public shares and maturation of public programmes differed widely.

Also worthy of note is the significance of the private sector. In at least seven countries, the private sector accounts for over 25 per cent of health expenditures. Thus, while analyses based only on public spending may provide useful information about government budgets, they will not provide a complete picture of overall health expenditures for a significant number of countries. Clearly, private sector financing and ownership are important aspects of most OECD health systems, and may become more important as countries attempt to reconcile access and new technologies with demographic and economic constraints.

Table 18

PUBLIC AND TOTAL HEALTH EXPENDITURES, 1960-1984
(Percent)

Country	1960		1965		1970		1975		1980		1982		1984	
	PH/TH	TH/GDP	PH/TH	TH/GDP	PH/TH	TH/GDP	PH/TH	TH/GDP	PH/TH	TH/GDP	PH/TH	TH/GDP	PH/TH	TH/GDP
Australia	47.6	5.2	54.0	5.3	55.8	5.7	73.8	7.6	62.5	7.4	62.1	7.5	84.5	7.8
Austria	65.3	4.4	64.7	4.7	59.1	5.3	60.8	6.4	62.3	7.0	61.1	7.3	60.9	7.2
Belgium	61.6	3.4	75.3	3.9	87.0	4.0	80.9	5.4	87.4	6.1	92.3	6.1	91.6	6.2
Canada	43.1	5.5	50.3	6.1	70.2	7.2	76.6	7.4	74.4	7.3	74.2	8.2	74.4	8.4
Denmark	88.7	3.6	85.9	4.8	86.3	6.1	91.9	6.5	85.2	6.8	85.6	6.9	83.4	6.3
Finland	54.5	4.1	64.3	4.8	72.1	5.6	78.6	6.1	78.2	6.3	79.7	6.6	78.8	6.6
France	57.8	4.3	68.1	5.3	71.7	6.1	72.2	7.6	72.0	8.5	71.1	9.3	71.2	9.1
Germany	67.5	4.7	70.9	5.1	74.2	5.5	80.2	7.8	79.3	7.9	78.7	8.1	78.2	8.1
Greece	57.9	2.9	71.1	3.1	53.9	4.0	61.6	4.0	83.9	4.2	84.4	4.4	79.3	4.6
Iceland	40.0	5.7	46.2	5.9	47.4	8.5	58.4	11.0	82.6	6.9	82.9	7.7	82.7	7.9
Ireland	76.0	4.0	76.2	4.4	77.8	5.6	82.5	7.7	93.5	8.5	93.6	8.1	86.9	8.0
Italy	83.1	3.9	87.8	4.6	86.4	5.5	86.1	6.7	87.8	6.8	84.6	7.2	84.1	7.2
Japan	60.4	3.0	61.4	4.3	69.8	4.4	72.0	5.5	70.8	6.4	70.3	6.8	72.1	6.6
Luxembourg						4.8			94.8	5.9		6.7		6.4
Netherlands	33.3	3.9	68.7	4.4	84.3	6.0	76.5	7.7	78.6	8.2	80.2	8.6	78.3	8.6
New Zealand							82.6	5.2	83.5	5.7	87.6	5.7	78.4	5.6
Norway	77.8	3.3	80.9	3.9	91.6	5.0	96.2	6.7	98.4	6.8	97.7	6.8	88.8	6.3
Portugal							58.9	6.4	68.9	5.9	71.1	5.7	71.1	5.5
Spain			52.6	2.7	54.7	4.1	70.4	5.1	73.5	5.9	72.4	6.3	72.3	5.8
Sweden	72.6	4.7	79.5	5.6	86.0	7.2	90.2	8.0	92.0	9.5	91.8	9.7	91.4	9.4
Switzerland		3.3			60.8	3.8	66.5	5.2	65.4	7.1		7.2		7.8
United Kingdom	85.2	3.9	85.8	4.1	87.0	4.5	90.3	5.6	90.4	5.6	90.2	5.7	88.9	5.9
United States	24.7	5.3	26.2	6.1	37.0	7.6	42.5	8.6	42.5	9.5	42.1	10.5	41.4	10.7
Mean*	61.0	4.2	67.6	4.8	72.1	5.8	76.2	7.0	79.0	7.2	79.0	7.5	78.7	7.5
High/low*	3.6	2.0	3.4	2.0	2.5	1.9	2.3	2.8	2.3	2.3	2.3	2.4	2.2	2.3
Standard deviation*	18.2	0.8	15.8	0.8	15.8	1.2	13.6	1.5	13.6	1.3	13.9	1.5	12.2	1.5
Mean - Big Seven	60.3	4.4	64.4	5.1	70.9	5.8	74.3	7.0	73.9	7.4	73.0	8.0	72.9	8.0

Notes: PH = Public Health Expenditure; TH = Total Health Expenditure; GDP = Gross Domestic Product;
  * Excludes Luxembourg, New Zealand, Portugal, Spain and Switzerland.
  Figures for 1984 are preliminary estimates.

Source: Measuring Health Care 1960-1983, OECD, Paris, 1985.

Table 19

PUBLIC COVERAGE RATIOS FOR HOSPITAL CARE

	1960	1965	1970	1975	1980	1983
Australia	77	77	79	100	100	100
Austria	78	78	92	97	99	99
Belgium	58	86	98	98	98	98
Canada	68	100	100	100	100	100
Denmark	95	95	100	100	100	100
Finland	100	100	100	100	100	100
France	85	88	96	98	100	100
Germany	86	87	93	95	95	95
Greece	30	40	91	98	98	98
Iceland	-	-	-	100	100	100
Ireland	85	85	85	85	100	100
Italy	87	91	93	100	100	100
Japan	-	100	100	100	100	100
Luxembourg	100	100	100	100	100	100
Netherlands	71	71	86	88	88	88
New Zealand	100	100	100	100	100	100
Norway	100	100	100	100	100	100
Portugal	18	32	52	90	100	100
Spain	50	55	61	81	83	87
Sweden	100	100	100	100	100	100
Switzerland	72	82	89	94	97	97
United Kingdom	100	100	100	100	100	100
United States	22	25	40	40	40	40
Mean*	75.3	80.6	88.3	93.5	95.1	95.3
High/Low*	5.6	4.0	2.5	2.5	2.5	2.5
Standard deviation*	26.2	23.4	17.0	13.5	13.4	13.2

Note: * Excludes Iceland and Japan.

Source: Measuring Health Care 1960-1983, OECD, Paris, 1985, Table C.1.

Nominal Levels of Health Expenditure

There are also significant differences in absolute spending levels among countries. Table 20 contains per capita health expenditures and per capita GDP denominated in US$ using GDP PPPs for 1970 (19 countries) and 1984 (21 countries). In 1984 per capita health expenditures for the 19 OECD countries averaged $917 compared to an average of $213 in 1970. Thus, over the period average per capita OECD health spending increased in nominal terms at a compound annual rate of 11.0 per cent in PPP-adjusted dollars, about 1.2 times the rate of increase in nominal GDP. This relationship between per capita health expenditures and per capita GDP is analysed in Chapter 7 below.

With regard to individual countries, in 1984 per capita spending is estimated to be greater than $1 200 in Canada, Sweden and the United States, but less than $500 in Greece and Spain (and Portugal). In 1970 per capita spending exceeded $300 in Canada, Sweden and the United States, but was less than $150 in Belgium, Greece, Ireland, Japan and Spain. The highest rates of

Table 20

PER CAPITA HEALTH SPENDING AND GDP, 1970 AND 1984
(US$ at GDP PPPs, current prices)

Country	1970		1984		Compound Annual Rate of Growth 1970-1984	
	Total Health per capita	GDP per capita	Total Health per capita	GDP per capita	Total Health per capita	GDP per capita
Australia	$232	$4 040	$ 994	$12 679	11.0	8.5
Austria	163	3 056	818	11 345	12.2	9.8
Belgium	147	3 652	777	12 439	12.6	9.1
Canada	322	4 452	1 275	15 198	10.3	9.2
Denmark	252	4 147	841	13 310	9.0	8.7
Finland	183	3 280	806	12 217	11.2	9.8
France	223	3 685	1 145	12 643	12.4	9.2
Germany	220	3 993	1 079	13 265	12.0	9.0
Greece	70	1 756	287	6 300	10.6	9.6
Iceland	288	3 382	1 045	13 238	9.6	10.2
Ireland	122	2 196	622	7 795	12.3	9.5
Italy	171	3 093	725	10 093	10.9	8.8
Japan	141	3 189	818	12 419	13.4	10.2
Netherlands	232	3 881	1 011	11 710	11.1	8.2
New Zealand	-	-	595	10 601	-	-
Norway	191	3 083	965	15 367	12.3	12.2
Portugal	-	-	275	5 021	-	-
Spain	102	2 473	476	8 279	11.6	9.0
Sweden	359	4 976	1 445	15 434	10.5	8.4
United Kingdom	161	3 563	658	11 068	10.6	8.4
United States	366	4 826	1 637	15 357	11.3	8.6
Mean	213	3 706	917 (871)*	12 113 (11 703)	11.0**	8.8**
High/low	5.2	2.8	5.7 (6.0)	2.4 (3.1)		
Standard deviation	80.2	931	326 (343)	2 577 (2 904)		

Notes: * The average based on dividing total health expenditure for all countries by total population (e.g. not country weighted) exceeds $1 050.
** Compound annual rates of growth of OECD average per capita health expenditures and GDP.
( ) Arithmetic average of 21 countries.

Sources: Measuring Health Care 1960-1983, OECD, Paris, 1985.
Health expenditures for 1984 are estimates based on the same source documents and methodology used in Measuring Health Care 1960-1983.
Purchasing power parities and population statistics are from National Accounts, Main Aggregates, Volume I, OECD, Paris, 1986.

growth in per capita spending, after adjustment for differences in international prices, were in Belgium, Japan, Norway and Ireland, while the lowest were in Denmark, Iceland and Canada. Nevertheless, the rank ordering of spending has not changed much since 1970.

Real Growth in Health Expenditures Relative to GDP

Changes in real resource commitments to health services within individual countries can also be compared by analysing changes in real health expenditures relative to real GDP, where both health expenditures and GDP are denominated in local currencies. While such information cannot be used to compare real quantities of health services across countries, it does measure the changes in real health resource commitments relative to real GDP within countries, and provides a basis for comparing these internal changes in real resource commitments across countries.

Table 21 contains the elasticities of real total health spending relative to real GDP. Real health spending and real GDP are calculated by dividing the nominal figures by the medical price index and the GDP deflator,

Table 21

REAL ELASTICITIES OF TOTAL HEALTH EXPENDITURES TO GDP, 1960-75, 1975-84, 1980-84, 1960-84

Country	1960-75	1975-84	1980-84	1960-84
Australia	0.8	0.6	1.0	0.9
Austria	0.7	0.7	0.5	0.8
Belgium	1.3	1.5	0.9	1.6
Canada	1.6	1.3	1.1	1.5
Denmark	1.9	1.4	-0.3	1.8
Finland	2.0	0.9	0.5	1.8
France	1.6	2.6	0.4	1.9
Germany	1.2	0.9	0.1	1.3
Greece	1.8	1.8	3.4	1.7
Ireland (a)	2.3	0.9	-1.5	2.0
Italy	0.9	1.3	1.1	1.1
Japan	1.3	1.6	1.1	1.4
Netherlands (a)	1.5	0.5	-1.3	1.3
Norway	1.7	1.5	0.5	1.5
Spain (b)	1.7	2.1	-0.4	1.9
Sweden	2.4	1.6	0.02	2.7
United Kingdom	2.1	1.0	0.4	2.1
United States	1.8	1.2	0.9	1.7
Mean	1.6	1.3	0.5	1.6
High-Low	1.7	2.1	4.9	1.9
Standard deviation	0.5	0.5	1.1	0.5

Notes: Total health expenditures are deflated by the health care price index. GDP is deflated by the GDP deflator.

The elasticity for the overall period can be greater or less than the elasticities for the two subperiods if a major structural shift in the relationship has occurred between the two periods. In this case the slope of the logarithmic regression line, the elasticity, can be greater or less than the slopes for the two subperiods.

a) 1975-83, 1960-83;
b) 1964-75, 1964-84.

Sources: Same as Table 20.

56

respectively. The elasticities are calculated for the 1960-1984 period, as well as the 1960-1975, 1975-1984 and 1980-84 sub-periods, in order to compare increases in the expansive pre-oil shock era to the slow growth, post-oil shock period. The average elasticity of 1.6 for these 18 OECD countries exceeded one for the 1960-1984 period, as well as the 1960-1975 (1.6) and 1975-1984 (1.3) subperiods. Thus, real health spending increased 60 per cent faster than real GDP between 1960-1984 and between 1960-1975, and 30 per cent faster between 1975-1984. These figures are consistent with rapid growth over the entire period, but more rapid growth in the expansive pre-1975 period than in the post-1975 period of reduced economic growth and public health programme maturation.

In fact, growth in real health expenditure relative to GDP appears to have slowed in the 1980s. For 1980-1984, the elasticity fell to 0.5, indicating that real health expenditure increased only 50 per cent as fast as real GDP. In 13 of the 18 countries, the elasticity was less than 1.0 (or negative) for this period. With relatively low real GDP growth, this would appear to indicate that health spending is under control, at least in terms of its rate of increase relative to GDP (although not necessarily in terms of overall expenditure efficiency) in several countries. Nevertheless, it is too soon to know if this is a short-run or long-run phenomenon. Similarly, there is still substantial excess capacity in most systems in terms of hospital beds and physicians.

Also of interest is the fact that in a significant number of countries, the elasticity for the entire 1960-84 period is greater or less than the elasticities for the 1960-75 and 1975-84 subperiods. This can occur statistically when there has been a structural shift in the relationship between the two time periods. Such structural shifts in health spending relative to GDP may have occurred in a number of countries, as governments, in reacting to the fiscal pressures resulting from the oil crises, limited health spending increases.

Decomposition of Nominal Health Expenditure Increases into Price, Population, and Utilisation and Intensity Effects

Aggregate increases in nominal health care expenditures can also be analysed in terms of increases in prices, population, and real benefits per person. In particular, increases in aggregate nominal health expenditures are disaggregated into health care inflation in the economy, overall inflation, health care inflation in excess of overall inflation, increases in population, and increases in average real benefits per person. Average real benefits per capita is the residual after adjusting nominal expenditures for price and population growth. This factor reflects all other factors not adequately controlled for by the price and population variables. For purposes of this analysis, this factor is called the utilisation and intensity effect.

This methodology is an identity (health expenditure growth equals health price growth x population growth x utilisation and intensity growth) and hence cannot be used to attribute causality. However, from a general health care policy perspective this methodology provides useful information about the relative magnitudes of general economic inflation, excess health care inflation, population growth, and growth in utilisation and intensity of services as the driving forces behind health care expenditure growth.

As this methodology is generally applied, the population factor is simply the increase in the number of people. It does not take account of changes in the age structure of the population. Hence, any expenditure growth resulting from population ageing is picked up by the utilisation and intensity (residual) factor. After discussing the results obtained from the usual decomposition methodology[1], the effects of ageing and population growth will be disaggregated through the use of a standardised population base.

Table 22 contains the disaggregation of increases in total health spending into price, population and utilisation and intensity effects for 20 OECD countries for 1960-1984. For these 20 countries, average nominal spending increased at a compound annual rate of 15.5 per cent, while health prices increased at 9.1 per cent, population at 0.8 per cent, and utilisation and intensity per person at 5.1 per cent. Average nominal spending for the seven major countries increased at a compound annual rate of 13.9 per cent. Health care prices increased at 7.0 per cent, population at 0.8 per cent and utilisation and intensity per person at 5.6 per cent. The data clearly suggest that the principal growth factors over the period are health care inflation and increases in utilisation and intensity of services per person with population growth being only a minor contributor.

Indeed much of the debate on controlling health care expenditures has focused on controlling prices. However, a somewhat different picture emerges when health care price inflation is compared with general economic inflation. Disaggregating health care price increases into general price increases and health care price increases in excess of overall inflation, general prices increased by 8.4 per cent, while health care price increases in excess of general price increases were only 0.6 per cent. Thus, general economic inflation, which can be considered as an exogenous influence on health spending, is the principal price effect, not excess health care inflation.

Within the health sector itself, the single largest endogenous factor affecting health expenditure growth is increases in utilisation and intensity of services per person. If general economic inflation is taken as given, increased utilisation and intensity of services per person combined with general economic inflation accounted for 13.9 percentage points of the 15.5 percentage point increase. The remainder of the increase is due to population growth and health care inflation in excess of

Table 22

DECOMPOSITION OF HEALTH EXPENDITURE INCREASES IN OECD COUNTRIES

	Nominal expenditure	GDP deflator	Health prices	Relative prices	Real expenditure	Of which	
						Demography	Utilisation/ intensity per person
	(Compound annual growth rates 1960-84)						
Canada	12.5	6.1	5.6	-0.5	6.5	1.4	5.1
France	15.3	7.5	6.9	-0.6	7.9	0.8	7.0
Germany	10.1	4.3	5.6	1.2	4.2	0.4	3.8
Italy	17.6	10.5	10.5	0.0	6.5	0.5	5.9
Japan	16.8	5.7	6.0	0.3	10.2	1.1	9.1
United Kingdom	13.1	8.7	8.3	-0.4	4.4	0.3	4.1
United States	11.8	5.1	6.2	1.0	5.3	1.1	4.1
Big 7 average *	13.9	6.8	7.0	0.1	6.4	0.8	5.6
Australia	13.7	7.2	9.5	2.2	3.8	1.6	2.1
Austria	11.3	5.1	8.3	3.0	2.8	0.3	2.5
Belgium	11.8	5.4	6.3	0.9	5.2	0.3	4.9
Denmark	14.1	8.2	8.2	0.0	5.4	0.5	5.0
Finland	15.4	8.8	8.1	-0.6	6.8	0.4	6.3
Greece	18.3	10.3	9.3	-1.0	8.3	0.7	7.5
Iceland	34.8	27.4	30.2	2.2	3.5	1.3	2.2
Ireland (a)	18.2	10.3	10.0	-0.3	7.5	0.9	6.6
Netherlands (a)	13.7	6.2	8.4	2.1	4.9	1.0	3.9
Norway	14.5	7.1	8.4	1.3	5.6	0.6	5.0
Spain (b)	21.8	12.1	13.0	0.8	7.7	1.0	6.7
Sweden	13.7	7.3	6.0	-1.2	7.3	0.5	6.8
Switzerland (c)	12.1	5.0	6.7	1.7	5.1	0.9	4.2
13 country average *	16.4	9.3	10.2	0.9	5.7	0.8	4.9
20 country average *	15.5	8.4	9.1	0.6	5.9	0.8	5.1

Notes: * Arithmetic average of relevant countries; a) 1960 - 1983; b) 1964 - 1984; c) 1960 - 1982.

Sources: Measuring Health Care 1960-1983, Paris, OECD, 1985 and OECD Secretariat estimates for 1984.

Table 23

POPULATION GROWTH AND AGEING, 1960-84
(Compound annual rate of growth)

	(A) Growth in Standardised Population	(B) Growth in Overall Population	(C) Growth in Utilisation/ Intensity	(D) Growth due to Ageing $(1 + A) / (1 + B)$	(E) Ageing-Adjusted Utilisation/ Intensity $(1 + C) / (1 + D)$
Canada	1.7	1.4	5.1	0.3	4.8
France	0.9	0.8	7.0	0.1	6.9
Germany	0.6	0.4	3.8	0.2	3.6
Italy	0.7	0.5	5.9	0.2	5.7
Japan	1.6	1.1	9.1	0.5	8.6
United Kingdom	0.6	0.3	4.1	0.3	3.8
United States	1.4	1.1	4.1	0.3	3.8
Big Seven Average	1.1	0.8	5.6	0.3	5.3
Australia	1.8	1.6	2.1	0.2	1.9
Belgium	0.4	0.3	4.9	0.1	4.8
Denmark	0.7	0.5	5.0	0.2	4.8
Finland	1.1	0.4	6.3	0.7	5.6
Ireland (a)	0.9	0.9	6.6	0.0	6.6
Netherlands (a)	1.4	1.0	3.9	0.4	3.5
Sweden	1.0	0.5	6.8	0.5	6.3
Switzerland (b)	1.2	0.9	4.2	0.3	3.9
Eight Country Average	1.1	0.8	5.0	0.3	4.7
Fifteen Country Average	1.1	0.8	5.3	0.3	5.0

Notes: a) 1960-1983.
        b) 1960-1982.

general economic inflation. Clearly, the hospital prospective payment systems in the United States and France and expenditure limits on physicians such as those in two Canadian provinces and in the 1977 German Cost Containment Act, as well as limitations imposed by several countries on their lists of reimbursable pharmaceuticals are attempts to deal with the utilisation and intensity issue.

The decomposition of health spending for individual countries mirrors the overall pattern with all countries experiencing substantial growth in real per capita benefits over the 1960-1984 period. From the perspective of health care inflation relative to overall inflation, the picture is somewhat more varied. While health care inflation exceeds overall inflation in eleven of the 20 countries, in nine countries overall inflation actually equalled or exceeded health care inflation. Analyses of this type performed for more recent time periods, such as 1975-84, also indicate that in a number of countries, excess health care price inflation would not appear to be a significant problem[2].

One can also analyse somewhat crudely the effects of past population growth and population ageing on past expenditure growth. To disaggregate the ageing effect from the utilisation and intensity factor and incorporate it into the population component, a standardised population is created for both the base and end years. To create this population, the expenditure weights in Chapter 8 are used. These weights provide the ratio of health spending for those 65 and over to those under 65. Using these weights, each aged person in both the base year (1960) and the end year (1984) is counted as if he/she were equivalent to *n* people less than age 65, where *n* is the expenditure weight for the aged versus the non-aged for that country. Thus a standardised population is developed for both base and end years, and the measured growth in this standardised population reflects both increased numbers of people as well as more (or less) aged people[3].

Table 23 contains the calculated rate of growth of the age-standardised population as well as the simple growth rate in terms of numbers of people in the overall population from Table 22 for the 15 countries for which a standardised population could be calculated. The average standardised population for the 15 countries grew at a compound annual rate of 1.1 per cent, compared to 0.8 per cent for growth in numbers of people only. Thus, on average, ageing of populations only contributed 0.3 percentage points to a 14 percentage point growth in nominal expenditures between 1960-84 for these 15 countries.

Dividing the previously calculated utilisation and intensity effect by this ageing effect removes population ageing impacts from this residual. This adjusted utilisation and intensity effect is also displayed in Table 23. On average, the utilisation and intensity effect increase for these countries is reduced from 5.3 per cent annually to 5.0 per cent. As far as individual countries are concerned, ageing of population ranged from no effect in Ireland to 0.7 in Finland. In no country was it a major factor. In Chapter 8, the expenditure effects of future ageing and population growth over the next 30 and 50 years are analysed. In the following chapter, specific utilisation components underlying these aggregate expenditure figures are analysed.

NOTES AND REFERENCES

1. For a description of this methodology, see *Social Expenditure 1960-1990 Problems of Growth and Control*, OECD, Paris, 1985, p. 44; and George Schieber and Jean-Pierre Poullier, "Comparison of Health Expenditures in OECD Countries", in John Virgo (ed.), *Restructuring Health Policy: An International Challenge*, International Health Economics and Management Institute, Edwardsville, Illinois, 1986.

2. See Jean-Pierre Poullier, "From Risk Aversion to Risk Rating: Trends in OECD Health Care Systems", *International Journal of Health Planning and Management*, Vol. 2, Special Issue, 1987.

3. Better estimates could be obtained if detailed spending weights for the very young and very old were available.

Chapter 6

COMPOSITION OF HEALTH SPENDING

In order to analyse health expenditure levels and trends in a policy-relevant manner, it is necessary to analyse the composition of health expenditures in terms of the specific types of services purchased, the physical amounts of such services, and their respective prices. Such an analysis can provide the basis for understanding: which services account for the major part of health spending; how the composition of spending has changed over time; and whether the growth in prices and/or physical quantities are the principal factor(s) responsible for increased spending. Such disaggregate information can also be used to evaluate previous policies undertaken to control spending, as well as point up those areas where expenditure restraint policies could have large impacts on overall spending. If such information on utilisation (and health status) were available by income class, current levels of, and changes in, access and use by specific socio-economic groups also could be evaluated.

Unfortunately, to date, no one internationally consistent data base provides the necessary information to analyse health expenditure and utilisation trends in such a disaggregate manner. The present OECD data base provides expenditure and price information for institutional care, ambulatory care, pharmaceuticals, and other services. It also provides utilisation and supply information on hospitals, physicians, and pharmacists. Information on hospital and physician expenditures can be obtained from other sources, but the data are generally not comparable because of definitional differences, the frequent inclusion in hospital expenditures of inpatient physician services, and the difficulty of separating outpatient hospital spending from total hospital expenditures. Moreover, detailed breakdowns of private expenditures by type of services are generally not available[1]. Nevertheless, given the policy relevance of analysing health expenditures by type of service, this chapter describes the composition of spending using the broad but relatively consistent OECD expenditure categories, utilisation, and price information. These data are supplemented by data from other sources, generally for smaller groups of countries, in order to provide as complete a picture as possible on levels and

trends in the composition of services in terms of expenditures, prices and utilisation.

Table 24 contains information for the OECD countries on the composition of public health expenditures in terms of institutional care, ambulatory care, pharmaceuticals, and other services for 1970 and the early 1980s. Public, not total health expenditures are analysed, because the data are more complete. Table 25 contains information on the prices of these components, as well as overall health prices, consumer prices as measured by the private final consumption deflator, and the GDP deflator. These data indicate once again that excess medical care price inflation does not appear to have been a serious problem in a number of OECD countries, although the medical care price index on average appears to have increased slightly faster than consumer prices and the GDP deflator. Nevertheless, caution is needed in interpreting these results, given the methodological nuances inherent in the construction of the medical care price indices in a number of countries.

Institutional Expenditures

Institutional expenditures are the largest and fastest growing component of health spending. Hospital expenditures are by far the largest component of institutional spending, which also includes expenditures on hospital-based physicians, nursing homes, and other institutional health facilities. In the early 1980s, institutional expenditures accounted for over half of all health spending in OECD countries. Institutional spending has been the fastest growing component, increasing from 50.9 per cent of the total in 1970 to over 54 per cent in the early 1980s. Similarly, the prices of institutional services have increased faster than the prices for all other health components, consumer prices and the GDP deflator.

With respect to individual countries, public institutional expenditures in the early 1980s are the largest component in almost every country, varying from 21.0 per cent in Belgium (where the data include only basic room and board outlays) to 73.9 per cent in

Table 24

COMPOSITION OF PUBLIC HEALTH SPENDING, 1970 AND 1980s

Country	Institutional			Ambulatory		
	1970	1980s	1970-80s	1970	1980s	1970-80s
Australia	35.9	47.6 (83)	2.5	19.1	18.1 (83)	-0.4
Austria	21.8	25.3 (83)	1.2	25.2	20.3 (84)	-1.4
Belgium	17.2	21.0 (81)	2.0	39.2	37.7 (81)	-0.3
Canada	66.8	59.3 (84)	-0.8	19.0	21.2 (81)	1.1
Denmark	64.7	73.9 (84)	1.0	26.3	22.0 (84)	-1.2
Finland	63.5	55.2 (83)	-1.0	17.0	28.1 (83)	5.0
France	45.9	59.5 (84)	2.1	26.3	22.9 (81)	-1.2
Germany	41.6	43.0 (83)	0.3	32.2	25.5 (83)	-1.6
Greece	40.1	49.5 (82)	2.0	17.3	13.4 (82)	-1.9
Ireland	-	73.4 (83)	-	-	11.5 (82)	-
Italy	51.7	55.3 (84)	0.5	32.2	27.8 (83)	-1.1
Luxembourg	-	32.5 (82)	-	-	21.5 (82)	-
Netherlands	56.1	69.3 (84)	1.7	5.0	22.2 (81)	31.3
New Zealand	68.8	69.2 (80)	0.1	9.9	6.1 (83)	-3.0
Norway	74.4	69.9 (81)	-0.5	17.8 (74)	15.3 (81)	-2.0
Portugal	46.6	46.3 (83)	-	26.5	20.7 (83)	-1.7
Spain	-	42.5 (81)	-	16.8 (72)	16.7 (80)	-0.1
Sweden	69.5	72.6 (83)	0.3	6.9	10.2 (83)	3.7
Switzerland	-	55.2 (80)	-	-	-	-
Turkey	34.7	49.5 (84)	3.9	-	60.2 (81)	-
United Kingdom	56.3	59.7 (79)	0.7	13.8	11.2 (82)	-1.6
United States	61.0	62.4 (84)	0.2	12.4	15.1 (84)	1.6
Mean	50.9	54.2	0.9	20.2	21.3	1.4
High - Low	57.2	52.9	4.9	34.2	54.1	34.3
Standard Deviation	16.6	15.1	1.3	9.2	11.4	7.7

Country	Pharmaceutical			Other		
	1970	1980s	1970-80s	1970	1980s	1970-80s
Australia	16.9 (73)	6.2 (83)	-6.3	-	28.1 (83)	-
Austria	15.4	9.9 (84)	-2.6	37.6	44.7 (83)	1.5
Belgium	18.9	11.8 (81)	-3.4	24.7	29.5 (81)	1.8
Canada	0.3	2.7 (81)	72.7	13.9	11.5 (81)	-1.6
Denmark	4.6	4.8 (83)	0.3	-	-	-
Finland	6.0	5.9 (84)	0.1	13.5	10.7 (83)	-1.6
France	20.8	13.1 (84)	-2.6	-	7.9 (81)	-
Germany	18.2	19.2 (83)	0.4	8.0	12.3 (83)	4.1
Greece	19.1	14.8 (82)	-1.9	23.5	22.3 (82)	-0.4
Ireland	2.7 (72)	7.0 (82)	15.9	-	9.7 (82)	-
Italy	16.0	13.0 (84)	-1.3	0.1	4.6 (83)	-
Netherlands	6.6	7.2 (84)	0.6	32.3	3.7 (81)	-8.0
New Zealand	13.5	12.3 (84)	-0.6	7.8	12.3 (80)	5.8
Norway	7.9 (74)	7.2 (81)	-1.3	-	7.6 (81)	-
Portugal	15.6	20.3 (83)	2.3	11.3	12.7 (83)	1.0
Spain	36.8 (72)	15.8 (83)	-5.2	-	25.7 (80)	-
Sweden	4.8	4.9 (83)	0.2	18.8	12.3 (83)	-2.7
Turkey	-	10.8 (83)	-	-	-	-
United Kingdom	9.9	10.3 (82)	0.3	20.0	20.0 (79)	-
United States	1.7	1.5 (84)	-0.8	24.9	21.0 (84)	-1.1
Mean	12.4	9.9	3.5	18.2	16.5	-0.1
High - Low	36.5	18.8	79.0	37.5	41.0	13.8
Standard Deviation	8.9	5.2	17.3	10.5	10.5	3.5

Source: Measuring Health Care 1960-1983, OECD, Paris, 1985, Tables A.2, A.4, A.6, A.8.
Figures for 1984 are estimates based on same sources and methodology.

Denmark, with an OECD average of 54.2. In 1970, institutional expenditures averaged 50.9 per cent, ranging from 17.2 in Belgium to 74.4 in Norway. Over this period Australia, France and Turkey experienced the largest growth in their institutional spending. In all but three countries, prices for institutional services were the fastest growing health price component, ranging from compound annual increases between 1970 and the early 1980s of 6.1 per cent in Japan to over 60 per cent in Italy and Greece. Furthermore, institutional health care price increases exceeded overall consumer prices and the GDP deflator by about 40 per cent. Only in four countries did institutional price inflation not exceed overall inflation.

Hospitals are the largest sub-component of institutional services. Due to a lack of standardisation of

Table 25

OVERALL AND MEDICAL CARE PRICE TRENDS
(Average annual increases 1970-84)

Country	Consumer prices	GDP deflator	Medical price index	Institutional	Ambulatory	Pharmaceutical
Australia	21.5	20.8	31.8	30.0 (83)	20.3 (83)	13.8 (83)
Austria	9.1	9.2	16.8	25.1	16.2	5.4
Belgium	10.7	11.6	12.0	17.0	13.3	4.3
Canada	15.0	13.6	13.1	22.0 (82)	12.0	12.6
Denmark	18.1	20.0	17.0	21.3	16.5	13.2
Finland	23.2	22.9	25.1	22.2	30.0 (83)	16.9 (83)
France	19.0	18.6	15.0	20.8	15.4	6.4
Germany	6.6	6.7	8.1	14.0 (82)	11.7 (82)	7.1
Greece	48.3	44.2	48.3	89.1 (82)	69.4 (82)	27.7
Ireland	35.7	37.8	36.0 (83)	29.0 (81)	29.0 (81)	26.3 (82)
Italy	43.0	42.8	36.4	68.7	37.4	14.0 (83)
Japan	8.7	11.0	7.8	6.1	6.1	7.2
Luxembourg	10.7	11.6	9.2 (82)	-	-	-
Netherlands	10.3	10.2	9.7 (83)	28.1	12.3	5.0
New Zealand	28.7	28.0	-	42.6 (83)	-	-
Norway	15.9	15.7	16.6	16.7	18.0	15.4
Portugal	62.5	71.5	-	62.5 (83)	62.9 (83)	22.5 (83)
Spain	39.9	40.8	42.5	-	-	7.2 (80)
Sweden	18.1	19.3	12.7	22.4 (80)	8.6 (83)	13.5
Switzerland	7.3	7.1	11.4	-	9.3 (83)	2.8 (83)
United Kingdom	27.8	26.1	27.7	39.6 (83)	-	23.0 (83)
United States	10.6	10.1	13.8	15.6	13.7	8.6
Mean*	19.6	19.6	20.0	28.0	20.6	12.3
High - Low*	41.7	37.5	40.5	83.0	63.3	23.4
Standard Deviation*	12.5	12.5	12.0	21.1	15.4	7.0
Mean - All countries	22.3	22.7	20.6	31.2	22.3	12.6

Notes: * Based on data for the 16 countries for which information on all components is readily available.

Source: Measuring Health Care 1960-1983, OECD, Paris, 1985.
Figures for 1984 are estimates based on same methodology and sources.

definitions, the aggregate nature of records in many administrative reporting systems, and basic differences in delivery systems, up-to-date strictly comparable expenditure and (to a lesser extent) utilisation data are not readily available. For example, many countries include nursing homes or long-term custodial care facilities in their hospital classification, while others have a separate classification. Other countries (e.g. the United Kingdom and Japan) provide extensive amounts of long-term care either in special long-term care hospitals or in separate wards of acute care hospitals. Many countries (the United Kingdom, Germany, Japan and Scandinavian countries) include the services of hospital-based physicians as part of the hospital service, while others (the United States, Belgium and Canada) classify such services as physician services. In some countries (Sweden, the United States, the Netherlands and the United Kingdom) extensive amounts of outpatient services are rendered in hospital clinics, while in others (Germany and Switzerland) virtually no outpatient care is performed in hospitals. Furthermore, there are no readily accessible data on expenditures, utilisation, and prices in acute care versus special care versus long-term care hospitals. Given these problems, caution is required in developing and interpreting hospital expenditure, price, and utilisation data.

Maxwell[2] attempted to standardize service classifications and derived data on health expenditures by type of service and source of payment for 1975 for 10 countries. The OECD attempted to develop standardized utilisation data for 1960-83 for inpatient medical care facilities. Hospital expenditure information from a variety of sources can be obtained for several countries.

Table 26 contains total hospital expenditures, PPP-adjusted per capita, per bed, per day (of utilisation), and per admission expenditures, as well as the hospital share of total health expenditures for 1982 for 14 OECD countries. These data are derived from different sources, and hence the definitions are not necessarily consistent. The data for all countries except the United States and Canada include expenditures for most hospital-based physician services (perhaps on the order of 15 per cent of the total). The expenditure data for all countries except France, Germany, Switzerland and Japan include expenditures on significant amounts of ambulatory care. The data for Australia, Canada, Ireland and Norway exclude capital expenditures (generally 4-15 per cent of the total). The data for Ireland are for public general hospitals, while the data for Australia are only for general hospitals. The data for Australia, Canada, Germany, France, Japan, the Netherlands, Switzerland and the United States are for total hospital expenditures, while the data for the United Kingdom, Ireland, Denmark, Finland, Iceland and Norway are only for publicly financed hospital expenditures. However, given the predominance of the public systems in these countries, large differences between public and total figures would not be expected. Furthermore, since the sources for the hospital expenditure data are sometimes different from those for the hospital bed and utilisation data, the expenditure figures may not be strictly consistent with the enumerated bed or utilisation figures.

The difficulties in developing a comparable hospital expenditure series can be illustrated by comparing the (public) percentage of hospital spending in the (public) total. If the individual country source data (and definitions) are used for both hospitals and all health expenditures, the percentage ranges from 33.7 per cent in Germany to 64.6 per cent in Denmark. Using the national accounts-based OECD figures of total (or public) health expenditures and the country source definitions of hospitals, the range is from 32.8 per cent in Japan to 70.4 in Denmark. Maxwell's 1975 ratios based

on his standardized definitions yield a range of from 35 per cent in Germany to 62.8 per cent in the United Kingdom.

These difficulties notwithstanding, the data indicate a 2.5 to 1 range in hospital expenditures per person, a 6.4 to 1 range in expenditures per bed, a 6 to 1 range in expenditures per day of utilisation, and a 3.6 to 1 range in expenditures per admission. Per capita expenditures ranged from under $300 per person in Japan ($230), Finland ($280) and Ireland ($260) to more than $500 per person in Iceland ($510), the Netherlands ($540), and the United States ($580). The 14-country OECD average is $410, and the coefficient of variation of 0.27, indicates much less dispersion in spending per capita than in spending per bed (0.50) and per day (0.47), and slightly less than spending per admission (0.34).

Expenditures per bed in 1982 varied from $19 000 in Japan to $122 000 in the United States with an OECD average of $50 000. However, if the highest and lowest two (e.g. the United States, Finland and Japan) are eliminated, the variation then is only 2 to 1, ranging from $34 000 in Germany to $65 000 in Canada.

Expenditures per hospital day varied from less than $100 per day in Finland ($70) and Japan ($60), to $360 per day in the United States with an OECD average of $170. As in the case of expenditures per bed if these

Table 26

HOSPITAL EXPENDITURES, 1982

Country	Total amount (millions of local currency units)	Amount per capita (PPPs)	Amount per bed (PPPs)	Amount per day (PPPs)	Amount per admission (PPPs)	Percent of all health expenditures		
						Country source	OECD	Maxwell (1975)
Australia (1) (2)	4 567	$310	$49 000	$200	$1 460	41.7	36.7	45.6
Canada (1)	12 470	450	65 000	210	3 020	41.4	41.4	53.8
Denmark (3)	19 340	490	63 000	220	2 590	64.6	70.4	–
Finland (3)	6 285	280	21 000	70	1 300	45.7	49.0	–
France	142 726	470	42 000	170	2 380	50.5	43.0	38.0
Germany	50 502	370	34 000	110	2 050	33.7	38.6	35.0
Iceland (3)	1 471	510	46 000	130	2 550	63.7	68.4	–
Ireland (1) (2) (3)	496	260	52 000	170	1 600	–	46.4	–
Japan	5 816 300	230	19 000	60	3 190*	41.9	32.8	–
Netherlands	18 841	540	45 000	140	4 640	59.5	59.0	52.6
Norway (1) (3)	11 186	410	61 000	220	2 800	45.6	45.3	–
Switzerland	6 751	470	37 000	125	3 300	46.3	44.4	44.9
United Kingdom (3)	8 912	320	39 000	140	2 490	61.7	61.5	62.8
United States	134 700	580	122 000	360	3 450	41.9	41.8	50.4
Mean		410	50 000	170	2 600			
High/Low		2.5	6.4	6.0	3.6			
Standard Deviation		110	25 000	80	890			

Notes: 1. Recurrent health expenditures; 2. General hospitals only; data on Ireland exclude private general hospitals; 3. Public expenditures.
  * Excludes clinic-based hospital beds.
  To assure as much correspondence as possible among costs, beds, and utilisation, the bed and utilisation statistics used here were taken from the same source as the hospital expenditure information whenever possible. As a result, they may differ from the figures presented in other tables based on the OECD data base.

Sources: Denmark, Finland, Iceland, Norway: Health Statistics in the Nordic Countries, 1982, 1983, 1984, Nordisk Medicinal - Statistisk Kommitté, Copenhagen, 1984, 1985, 1986. Norwegian expenditure data provided by Royal Norwegian Ministry of Health and Social Affairs.
France, Germany, the Netherlands, Switzerland, the United Kingdom: Eurocare, Health Service Consultants, Basle; and Annual Abstract of Statistics 1986 Edition, U.K. Central Statistical Office, London, 1986.
Australia: Australian Health Expenditure 1979-80 and 1981-82, Australian Institute of Health, Canberra, 1986, and data supplied by Australian Department of Health.
Canada: National Health Expenditures in Canada 1970-1982, Health and Welfare Canada, Ottawa; and Canada Yearbook 1985, Minister of Supply and Services, Ottawa, 1985.
United States: Health Care Financing Review, Fall 1985; Health United States 1985, National Center for Health Statistics, Hyattsville, Maryland, 1985; and Statistical Abstract of the United States, 1985, U.S. Bureau of the Census, Washington, D.C., 1984.
Ireland: Statistical Information Relevant to the Health Services, 1983, 1984, Department of Health, prepared by the Planning Unit, Dublin.
Japan: Japanese Medical Care Expenditure, Statistics and Information Department of the Japanese Ministry of Health and Welfare, Tokyo, 1983; and Hospital Survey 1983, Japanese Ministry of Health and Welfare, Tokyo, 1986.
Measuring Health Care 1960-83, OECD, Paris, 1985.
National Accounts Main Aggregates Volume 1, OECD, Paris, 1986.
Robert J. Maxwell, Health and Wealth: An International Study of Health Care Spending, Lexington Books, Lexington, Mass., 1981.

extreme values are dropped, there is substantially less variation among the remaining 11 countries, with expenditures per day varying from $110 per day in Germany to $220 in Denmark and Norway.

Expenditures per admission varied from $1 600 or less per admission in Finland ($1 300), Australia ($1 460) and Ireland ($1 600) to more than $3 400 in the Netherlands ($4 640) and the United States ($3 450) with a 14-country OECD average of $2 600. However, if these extreme values are dropped the variation is about 1.6 to 1, ranging from $2 050 in Germany to $3 300 in Switzerland.

Nevertheless, these differences in expenditures per admission mask enormous differences in average lengths of stay per admission. For example, as discussed below in detail, the average lengths of stay in Germany are almost double those in the United States, while those in Japan are 5 times greater. Yet, the expenditures per admission are substantially higher in the United States. While some of these differences can be explained by lack of comparability of hospital service definitions (e.g. inclusion of lower cost long-term care beds) and hence differences in casemix, as shown below substantial differences in average length of stay still persist after adjustment for casemix. Thus, it would appear that a significant proportion of these differences in costs are due to differences in intensity of services per case, efficiency, and possibly outcomes. However, certain studies have shown that large differences in length of stay within given countries are not necessarily related to differences in health outcomes[3]. This raises the question of whether substantial savings could be achieved by reducing lengths of stay without concomitant increases in intensity of services offsetting the potential savings from the reductions in lengths of stay. While it is difficult to definitively answer this question, the large documented differences in medical practice, inappropriate use of certain procedures (e.g. cesearean versus normal deliveries, complete versus partial mastectomies, cardiac-by-pass surgery versus drug therapy), as well as documented savings from alternative reimbursement and delivery arrangements would suggest that significant savings could be achieved through reductions in lengths of stay[4].

However, these results must be heavily caveated. While certain differences can be explained in terms of systems characteristics (tough planning rules in Finland, very limited outpatient hospital care in Germany, inclusion of salaries of hospital-based physicians in many countries), much of the variation is due to differences in medical practice, definitions, and types of service provided. For example, the low *per diem* and bed

Table 27

INPATIENT MEDICAL CARE BEDS PER 1 000 POPULATION, 1960, 1970, 1980s

| Country | 1960 | | 1970 | | 1980s | | Annual % of change | | |
							1960-70	1970-80s	1960-80s
Australia	9.0	(62)	9.9		11.0	(81)	1.3	1.0	1.2
Austria	10.3		10.5		10.8	(83)	0.2	0.2	0.2
Belgium	6.0		8.3		9.5	(82)	3.8	1.2	2.7
Canada	6.2		7.0		6.9	(82)	1.3	-0.1	0.5
Denmark	8.1	(61)	8.1		7.4	(83)	0	-0.7	-0.4
Finland	11.5		15.1		15.5	(82)	3.1	0.2	1.6
France	9.6	(62)	10.4	(72)	11.6	(83)	0.8	1.0	1.0
Germany	10.5		11.3		11.1	(82)	0.8	-0.1	0.3
Greece	5.8		6.2		6.2	(81)	0.7	0	0.3
Iceland	9.8		9.5		11.1	(82)	-0.3	1.4	0.6
Ireland	–		12.6		9.7	(80)		-2.3	
Italy	7.5		8.8		7.7	(83)	1.7	-1.0	0.1
Japan	7.4		10.2		12.1	(83)	3.8	1.4	2.8
Luxembourg	11.9		12.6		13.0	(83)	0.6	0.2	0.4
Netherlands	11.0		11.4		12.0	(83)	0.4	0.4	0.4
New Zealand	12.7		10.8		9.9	(83)	-1.5	-0.6	-1.0
Norway	9.3	(63)	8.3		6.5	(83)	-1.5	-1.7	-1.5
Portugal	5.3		6.0		5.1	(82)	1.3	-1.3	-0.2
Spain	4.3	(62)	4.7		5.4	(81)	1.2	1.4	1.3
Sweden	13.7		14.9		14.0	(83)	0.9	-0.5	0.1
Switzerland	12.6		11.2		11.5	(82)	-1.1	0.2	-0.4
Turkey	1.7		2.0		2.1	(82)	1.8	0.4	1.1
United Kingdom	10.3	(61)	9.4		8.1	(81)	-1.0	-1.3	-1.1
United States	9.2		7.9		5.9	(81)	-1.4	-2.3	-1.7
Mean	8.9		9.5		9.3		0.7	-0.1	0.4
Range	12.0		13.1		13.4		5.3	3.7	4.5
Standard Deviation	3.0		3.0		3.2		1.5	1.1	1.1

Note: Data for Ireland in this table include long-term hospitals.

Source: Measuring Health Care 1960-1983, OECD, Paris, 1985, Table D.4.

expenditures in Japan and the United Kingdom are in part due to significant amounts of long-term care being provided in hospitals instead of in nursing homes. Similarly, if outpatient hospital services were excluded, the cost per capita, per bed, per day, and per admission figures in a number of countries would be reduced (e.g. the United States per-day cost for inpatient hospital care is $327)[5]. Differences in staffing and the ages and amounts of equipment and physical plant will also have significant effects on expenditure differences. Differences in efficiency are also a major determinant of comparative expenditure differences, although not readily measurable with data at this level of aggregation. Differences in expenditures per capita, per bed, per day, and per admission, are also due to differences in number of beds per capita, use of services, occupancy rates, admission rates and lengths of stay.

As shown in Table 27, the number of hospital beds per 1 000 population grew between 1960 and 1970 but has on average declined slightly between 1970 and the early 1980s[6]. On average the number of beds per 1 000 increased from 8.9 in 1960 to 9.5 in 1970, but dropped slightly to 9.3 in the 1980s. Again there is variation among countries, but generally expansions of hospital sectors following the Second World War have been so successful that most OECD countries are now facing

excess hospital capacity. Indeed, as discussed below, half of the OECD countries have occupancy rates of less than 80 per cent.

With respect to individual countries, in 1960 beds per 1 000 capita ranged from less than 5 in Spain and Turkey to more than 10 in Austria, Finland, Germany, Luxembourg, the Netherlands, New Zealand, Sweden, Switzerland and the United Kingdom with an OECD average of 8.9 and a coefficient of variation of 0.34. By the 1980s the range was still from less than 5 in Turkey to more than 10 in some 11 countries with an average of 9.3 and a coefficient of variation of 0.34. Belgium and Japan had the largest increases in beds per capita over the period, on the order of 3 per cent annual increases, and Denmark, New Zealand, Norway, Portugal, Switzerland, the United Kingdom and the United States had decreases.

Per capita use of these inpatient medical care beds, as shown in Table 28, also varies significantly across countries, although OECD average utilisation per person has remained relatively constant at about 2.8 days per capita between 1960 and the early 1980s. In 1960, utilisation varied between less than 1 day per capita in Spain and Portugal to over four days in Finland and Sweden. In the early 1980s, utilisation per capita varied from less than two days in Greece, Ireland,

Table 28

INPATIENT DAYS PER CAPITA 1960, 1970, 1980s

Country	1960	1970	1980s	Annual % of change		
				1960-70	1970-80s	1960-80s
Australia	2.4 (63)	2.7	3.2 (81)	1.8	1.7	1.8
Austria	3.5	3.5	3.4 (83)	0	-0.2	-0.1
Belgium	1.6 (65)	2.3	2.8 (81)	8.8	2.0	4.7
Canada	1.8	2.0	2.1 (82)	1.1	0.4	0.8
Denmark	2.6	2.6	2.2 (82)	0	-1.3	-0.7
Finland	4.2	5.0	4.8 (83)	1.9	-0.3	0.6
France	2.6	3.4	3.1 (83)	3.1	-0.7	0.8
Germany	3.6	3.6	3.4 (82)	0	-0.5	-0.3
Greece	1.3	1.6	1.6 (82)	2.3	0	1.0
Iceland	3.4	3.6	3.9 (81)	0.6	0.8	0.7
Ireland			1.5 (82)			
Italy	2.2	2.6	2.2 (83)	1.8	-1.2	0
Japan	2.1	3.0	3.7 (83)	4.3	1.8	3.3
Luxembourg	3.4	3.6	3.7 (83)	0.6	0.2	0.4
Netherlands	3.8 (68)	3.8	4.0 (83)	0	0.4	0.4
New Zealand	3.3	3.0	2.7 (83)	-0.9	-0.8	-0.8
Norway	3.1	2.8	2.0 (81)	-1.0	-2.6	-1.7
Portugal	0.8	1.1	1.4 (81)	3.8	2.5	3.6
Spain	0.8 (66)	1.3	1.3 (81)	15.6	0	4.2
Sweden	4.3	4.5	4.8 (83)	0.5	0.5	0.5
Switzerland	3.9	3.4	3.1 (82)	-1.3	-0.7	-0.9
United Kingdom	3.4	2.9	2.4 (81)	-1.5	-1.6	-1.4
United States	2.8	2.3	1.7 (81)	-1.8	-2.4	-1.9
Mean	2.8	2.9	2.8	1.8	-0.1	0.7
Range	3.5	3.9	3.5	17.4	5.1	6.6
Standard Deviation	1.0	1.0	1.0	3.9	1.3	1.8

Sources: Measuring Health Care 1960-1983, OECD, Paris, 1985, Table D.1.
Data for Ireland are for public general hospitals which account for about half of all hospital beds (5.0 per thousand population). See Statistical Information relevant to the Health Services, 1983, 1984, Table G.1, prepared by the Planning Unit.

Portugal, Spain and the United States to four days or more in Finland, the Netherlands and Sweden. Over this period the largest average annual growth (in excess of 3 per cent) in utilisation took place in Belgium, Japan, Portugal and Spain. Utilisation fell in Austria, Denmark, Germany, New Zealand, Norway, Switzerland, the United Kingdom and the United States. Perhaps of more interest is the fact that utilisation per capita declined in half of the OECD countries between 1970-83, compared to only five between 1960-70.

Also of interest is the relationship between use and availability. Chart 9 shows the relationship in the early 1980s across countries of per capita days and per capita beds. There is a strong statistically significant positive relationship and a simple correlation of .94, which lends credence at an international level to the Roemer hypothesis linking bed availability to bed use[7]. However, it is plausible that demand side as opposed to (and/or in addition to) supply side factors have influenced use of available beds. Causality cannot be attributed based on the simple statistical relationships developed here.

Given the number of beds available, per capita use of services determines the occupancy rate. Per capita use and the occupancy rate also depend on the admission

Chart 9
PER CAPITA USE, BEDS PER CAPITA, 1983[a]

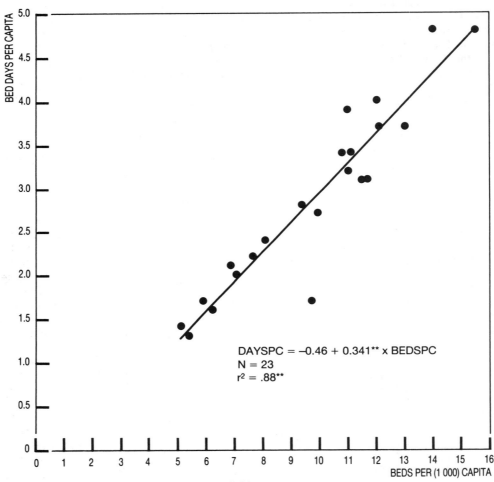

DAYSPC = −0.46 + 0.341** x BEDSPC
N = 23
r² = .88**

Notes : a. Data are for 1983 or nearest available years.
Excludes Turkey.
DAYSPC = Inpatient days per capita.
BEDSPC = Beds per 1 000 capita.
N = Number of countries.
r² = Adjusted correlation coefficient squared.
** = Statistically significant at .01 level.

Source : Same as Tables 27 and 28.

Table 29

HOSPITAL OCCUPANCY RATES, 1960, 1970, 1980s
(Percent)

Country	1960		1970	1980s		Annual % of change		
						1960-70	1970-83	1960-80s
Australia	71.5	(63)	74.5	79.5	(81)	0.6	0.6	0.6
Austria	92.9		91.2	86.6	(83)	-0.2	-0.4	-0.3
Belgium	68.5	(65)	75.6	81.6	(81)	2.1	0.7	1.2
Canada	79.7		78.6	83.3	(82)	-0.1	0.5	0.2
Denmark	88.2	(61)	87.7	78.6	(82)	-0.1	-0.9	-0.5
Finland	99.5		91.0	84.7	(82)	-0.9	-0.6	-0.7
France	91.2	(62)	88.2	73.2	(83)	-0.4	-1.3	-0.9
Germany	94.0		87.7	84.1	(82)	-0.7	-0.3	-0.5
Greece	61.4		70.7	71.2	(81)	1.5	0.1	0.8
Iceland	94.8		100.0	97.0	(81)	1.0	-0.6	0.1
Ireland				80.1	(82)			
Italy	80.6		81.1	78.1	(83)	0.1	-0.3	-0.1
Japan	78.1		80.3	83.8	(83)	0.3	0.3	0.3
Luxembourg	78.4		78.1	78.4	(83)	-0.03	0.03	0.0
Netherlands	92.3	(68)	91.5	91.5	(83)	-0.4	0.0	-0.1
New Zealand	77.3		76.4	74.8	(83)	-0.1	-0.2	-0.1
Norway	91.2	(63)	92.9	77.5	(81)	0.3	-1.5	-0.8
Portugal				74.5	(81)			
Spain			76.4	66.0	(81)		-1.2	
Sweden	86.0		82.7	94.0	(83)	-0.4	1.0	0.4
Switzerland	84.7		83.6	73.7	(82)	-0.1	-0.1	-0.6
United Kingdom	90.1		84.1	81.4	(81)	-0.7	-0.3	-0.4
United States	83.6		80.0	78.6	(81)	-0.4	-0.2	-0.3
Mean	84.2		83.4	80.5		0.07	-0.2	-0.1
Range	38.1		29.3	31.0		3.0	2.5	2.1
Standard Deviation	9.8		7.4	7.2		0.7	0.7	0.6

Source: Calculated from sources in Tables 27 and 28. Hospital occupancy rate = (Days per capita x population) / (365 x hospital beds)

rate and average length of stay (ALOS). Differences in these parameters can have significant effects on hospital costs. Although countries with different admission rates and lengths of stay can still have the same per capita utilisation in terms of days, their costs could be quite different, since shorter stays are generally associated with higher costs per day, *ceteris paribus*, given the higher intensity of services (diagnostic tests, emergency procedures, etc.) generally performed at the beginning of the stay.

Table 29 contains occupancy rates for 1960, 1970 and the early 1980s. Occupancy rates have been falling slightly over the entire period with the largest declines taking place in the past 10 years. The average OECD occupancy rate has declined from 84.2 in 1960 to 80.5 in the 1980s. Half of the countries have experienced declines in their occupancy rates over this period. The largest declines took place in Finland, France and Norway, while the largest increases took place in Belgium and Greece. In the early 1980s occupancy rates varied from less than 70 per cent in Spain to over 90 per cent in Iceland, the Netherlands and Sweden. For the major seven OECD countries the rates varied from 73.2 in France to 84.1 in Germany with an average of 80.5.

Roemer's Law suggests that there should be a direct (positive) relationship between bed availability and the occupancy rate. On the other hand, an inverse relationship is possible if countries are facing severe bed shortages, that is all available beds would tend to be occupied. Chart 10 displays the relationship between the number of beds per capita and the occupancy rate. A positive statistically significant relationship is found with a simple correlation of 0.55. Thus, it would appear that despite an oversupply of beds in many OECD countries, those countries with higher per capita bed availability have higher occupancy rates, and, as previously shown, higher per capita use.

Admission rates provide a measure of hospital turnover. They also provide an indication, holding other factors constant, about whether hospital use is of a short-term acute care or long-term chronic care nature. As shown in Table 30, admission rates, defined as the percentage of population admitted, have increased steadily between 1960 and the early 1980s in virtually every country. The OECD average admission rate increased from 10.4 per cent of population in 1960 to 12.5 in 1970 to 15.3 per cent in the early 1980s. This indicates greater accessibility and use of hospital services. Admission rates increased the most in Australia,

Chart 10

OCCUPANCY RATES, BEDS PER CAPITA, 1983[a]

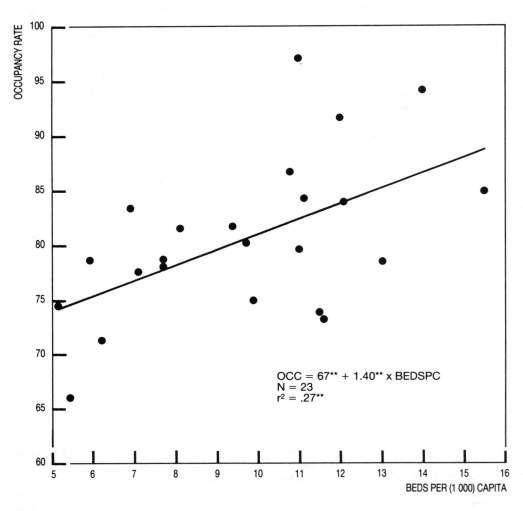

Notes : a. Data are for 1983 or nearest available years.
Same as Chart 9.
OCC = Occupancy rate.

Source : Same as Tables 27 and 29.

Belgium, France, Iceland, Italy, Japan, New Zealand and Portugal, and the least in Canada, Switzerland and the United States, where they were already high. In the early 1960s admission rates ranged from under 5 per cent in Japan and Portugal to over 14 per cent in Austria and Canada. In the 1980s admission rates were under 9 per cent only in Japan and above 20 per cent in Australia, Austria, Finland and Iceland.

Average lengths of stay data are displayed in Table 31. These figures are quite sensitive to the types of facilities included in the category "hospital". While there are undoubtedly legitimate differences in lengths of stay due to differences in illness patterns, intensity of services (including capital equipment and hospital staff per bed), medical practice, efficiency, etc., it is clear that a large, albeit not quantifiable, part of the differences observed in this table are due to the inclusion of long-term care facilities in the hospital classification of a number of countries. Thus, these data should be interpreted with extreme caution.

Average lengths of hospital stay (ALOS) have been falling steadily since 1960 in all OECD countries except Canada. The OECD ALOS fell from 26.3 days in 1960, to 22.2 in 1970 to 17.9 in the 1980s, an annual average

Table 30

HOSPITAL ADMISSION RATES, 1960, 1970, 1980s
(Percent of population)

Country	1960	1970	1980s	Annual % of change		
				1960-70	1970-80s	1960-80s
Australia	12.5 (61)	17.5	21.0 (80)	4.4	2.0	3.6
Austria	14.1	15.6	20.7 (83)	1.1	2.5	2.0
Belgium	8.0 (65)	9.3	13.9 (81)	3.3	4.5	4.6
Canada	15.0	16.5	14.7 (82)	1.0	-0.9	-0.1
Denmark	12.7 (63)	14.4	19.2 (83)	1.9	2.6	2.6
Finland	13.1	18.2	20.9 (83)	3.9	1.1	2.6
France	6.7 (66)	7.4	11.8 (83)	2.6	4.6	4.5
Germany	12.5	14.6	18.1 (82)	1.7	2.0	2.0
Greece	7.0 (61)	10.5	11.9 (82)	5.6	1.1	3.3
Iceland	11.8 (63)	16.2	20.2 (82)	5.3	2.1	3.7
Ireland			16.4 (82)			
Italy	7.8	13.8	15.4 (83)	7.7	0.9	4.2
Japan	3.7	5.4	6.7 (83)	4.6	1.9	3.5
Luxembourg	11.6	13.4	18.1 (83)	1.6	2.7	2.4
Netherlands	8.6 (63)	10.0	11.8 (83)	2.3	1.4	1.9
New Zealand	7.9	9.3	15.7 (83)	1.8	5.3	4.3
Norway	11.7 (63)	13.2	14.9 (83)	1.8	1.0	1.4
Portugal	4.2	5.9	9.6 (82)	4.0	5.2	5.8
Spain	~	7.1 (72)	9.2 (81)		3.3	
Sweden	13.4	16.6	19.2 (83)	2.4	1.2	1.9
Switzerland	12.4	13.1	12.8 (82)	0.6	-0.2	0.1
United Kingdom	9.2	11.3	12.7 (81)	2.3	1.1	1.8
United States	13.9	15.5	17.0 (81)	1.2	0.9	1.1
Mean	10.4	12.5	15.3	2.9	2.1	2.7
Range	11.3	12.8	14.3	7.1	6.2	5.9
Standard Deviation	3.3	3.9	4.1	1.8	1.6	1.5

Source: Measuring Health Care 1960-1983, OECD, Paris, 1985, Table D.1(A).

Table 31

AVERAGE LENGTH OF STAY, 1960, 1970, 1980s

Country	1960	1970	1980s	Annual % of change		
				1960-70	1970-80s	1960-80s
Australia	9.8 (67)	8.9	7.4 (80)	-3.1	-1.7	-1.9
Austria	24.8	22.2	16.3 (83)	-1.0	-2.0	-1.5
Belgium	14.4 (65)	15.6	13.5 (81)	1.7	-1.2	-0.4
Canada	11.1	11.5	13.3 (82)	0.4	1.3	0.9
Denmark	22.2 (63)	18.1	11.9 (82)	-2.6	-2.9	-2.4
Finland	31.7	27.3	22.2 (82)	-1.4	-1.6	-1.4
France	22.8 (61)	18.3	14.1 (83)	-2.2	-1.8	-1.7
Germany	28.7	24.9	18.7 (82)	-1.3	-2.1	-1.6
Greece	18.8 (61)	15.0	13.0 (82)	-2.2	-1.1	-1.5
Iceland	30.0 (63)	28.8	18.0 (82)	-0.6	-3.1	-2.1
Ireland	~	13.3	9.0 (82)		-2.7	
Italy	27.9	18.8	12.0 (83)	-3.3	-2.8	-2.5
Japan	57.3	55.3	55.1 (83)	-0.3	-0.02	-0.2
Luxembourg	29.0	27.0	21.0 (83)	-0.7	-1.7	-1.2
Netherlands	39.4 (68)	38.2	34.1 (83)	-1.5	-0.9	-1.0
New Zealand	18.9	15.4 (71)	12.4 (83)	-1.7	-1.6	-1.5
Norway	26.3 (63)	21.0	13.0 (81)	-2.9	-3.5	-2.8
Portugal	19.5	18.4	14.4 (81)	-0.6	-2.0	-1.2
Spain		18.0 (72)	14.6 (81)	14.6		-2.1
Sweden	31.8	27.2	22.7 (83)	-1.4	-1.3	-1.2
Switzerland	31.7	26.0	25.4 (82)	-1.8	-0.2	-0.9
United Kingdom	35.9	25.7	18.6 (81)	-2.8	-2.5	-2.3
United States	20.5	14.9	9.9 (81)	-2.7	3.1	-2.5
Mean	26.3	22.2	17.9	-1.5	-1.5	-1.5
Range	47.5	46.4	47.7	5.0	6.6	3.7
Standard Deviation	10.5	9.9	10.1	1.2	1.5	0.9

Source: Measuring Health Care 1960-1983, OECD, Paris, Table D.1(B).

percentage decline of 1.5 per cent. In 1960, ALOS varied from less than 15 days in Australia, Belgium and Canada to 30 or more days in Finland, Iceland, Japan, the Netherlands, Sweden, Switzerland and the United Kingdom. By the 1980s, ALOS exceeded 25 days only in Japan, the Netherlands and Switzerland, while ALOS was less than 15 days in Australia, Belgium, Canada, Denmark, France, Greece, Ireland, Italy, New Zealand, Norway, Portugal, Spain and the United States. The data indicate quite clearly both the significant downward trend and the significant reduction in the range and variability of the distribution.

As stated previously, shorter lengths of stay may be associated with greater intensity of services per day. If employees per bed are taken as a proxy measure of intensity, ALOS would be expected to be inversely associated with numbers of hospital employees per bed, the more employees the greater the intensity of service, the shorter the stay. An inverse relationship is found with a correlation of -0.39, but the relationship is not statistically significant[8]. ALOS is also found to vary directly with hospital beds per capita. It would be expected, *ceteris paribus*, that the smaller the number of beds per capita, the shorter the stay. In other words, fewer beds per capita, *ceteris paribus*, would imply greater demand per bed, and hence pressure to free up occupied beds as soon as possible. The data in Chart 11 show the expected direct relationship which is statistically significant with a simple correlation of 0.48. It might also be hypothesized that lengths of stay are

Chart 11

AVERAGE LENGTH OF STAY, BEDS PER CAPITA, 1983[a]

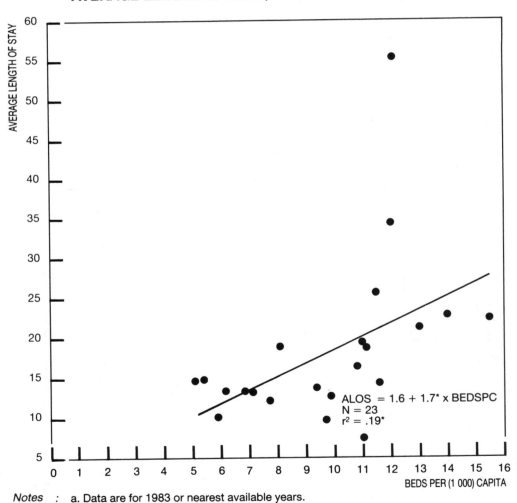

$$ALOS = 1.6 + 1.7^* \times BEDSPC$$
$$N = 23$$
$$r^2 = .19^*$$

Notes : a. Data are for 1983 or nearest available years.
Same as Chart 9.
ALOS = Average length of stay.
* = Statistically significant at .05 level.

Source : Same as Tables 27 and 31.

70

inversely related with occupancy rates, the higher the occupancy rate, the shorter the length of stay. However, a positive relationship is also plausible, if a significant number of beds are long-term care beds with little turnover (e.g. high occupancy rates and long lengths of stay). A positive but not statistically significant correlation of 0.36 is found.

These differences in length of stay may also be related to differences in the casemix of patients. Table 32 displays average lengths of stay in somatic hospitals for the major seven OECD countries for 18 ICD disease classifications. The differences are large. Indeed, given the enormous differences between Japan and all other countries, it would appear that essentially different types of institutions are being compared. Thus, the Japanese data are excluded from the summary statistics. However, even excluding Japan, in almost all cases the ranges indicate at least a 2.5:1 difference between

Table 32

MEAN LENGTH OF STAY IN SOMATIC HOSPITALS
(in days) - 1980

International classification of disease categories	Canada (1978)	France (1978)	Germany	Italy	Japan	United Kingdom	United States	Mean*	High/ Low*	Standard deviation*	Coefficient of variation*
Infectious and parasitic diseases (001-139)	7.7	16.7	17.9	26.1	117.6	11.0	6.9	14.4	3.8	7.3	0.51
Neoplasms (140-239)	14.8	11.3	18.9	17.7	51.7	14.5	10.5	14.6	1.8	3.3	0.23
Endocrine and metabolic diseases (240-279)	14.9	17.4	22.2	16.8	51.9	18.2	9.6	16.5	2.3	4.2	0.25
Diseases of the blood (280-289)	10.8	15.6	18.4	13.7	41.7	11.9	7.2	12.9	2.6	3.9	0.30
Mental disorders (290-319)	19.9	17.5	38.3	87.1	333.3	49.9	11.6	37.4	7.5	28.3	0.76
Diseases of the nervous system (320-389)	..	14.4	18.5	17.3	86.4	36.3	5.4	18.4	6.7	11.3	0.61
Diseases of the circulatory system (390-459)	20.2	19.8	23.5	18.7	100.4	..	10.0	18.4	2.4	5.0	0.27
Diseases of the respiratory system (460-519)	6.9	13.0	13.7	11.7	25.6	14.4	6.3	11.0	2.3	3.5	0.32
Diseases of the digestive system (520-579)	8.7	13.6	17.2	13.5	32.6	9.4	7.0	11.6	2.5	3.8	0.33
Diseases of the genito-urinary system (580-629)	7.1	10.6	14.2	11.3	31.0	10.3	5.6	9.9	2.5	3.1	0.31
Complications of pregnancy and childbirth (630-676)	5.0	6.6	9.1	7.0	8.7	..	2.5	6.0	3.6	2.5	0.41
Diseases of the skin and subcutaneous tissue (680-709)	9.0	13.4	20.4	11.3	22.6	13.2	8.0	12.6	2.6	4.4	0.35
Diseases of musculo-skeletal system & connective tissue (710-739)	12.7	19.2	23.4	14.7	72.6	17.6	8.3	16.0	2.8	5.3	0.33
Congenital anomalies (740-759)	10.7	13.3	16.2	11.6	37.7	10.4	6.6	11.5	2.5	3.2	0.28
Certain causes of perinatal morbidity and mortality (760-779)	6.8	18.8	20.3	13.9	12.5	8.6	8.7	12.9	2.3	5.7	0.45
Symptoms of ill-defined conditions (780-799)	7.5	11.6	16.5	11.4	17.5	..	4.5	10.3	3.7	4.6	0.44
Accidents, poisoning and violence (800-999)	9.6	10.5	17.8	8.2	37.5	10.6	7.7	10.7	2.3	3.7	0.34
All other	6.3	7.8	..	9.2	0.9	..	3.7	6.8	2.5	2.4	0.35
All categories (001-999)	10.7	13.5	18.4	15.4	55.1	13.3	7.3	13.1	2.5	3.8	0.29

Note: * Excludes Japan.

Source: Measuring Health Care 1960-1983, OECD, Paris, 1985, Table E.2.

Table 33

MEAN LENGTH OF STAY IN SOMATIC HOSPITALS BY I.C.D. SUB-CATEGORIES
(in days) - 1980

International classification of disease categories	Canada (1978)	France (1978)	Germany	Italy	Japan	United Kingdom	United States	Mean*	High/ Low*	Standard deviation*	Coefficient of variation*
Pulmonary tuberculosis (011)	34.0	32.8	19.4	85.8	..	37.6	12.8	37.1	6.7	25.7	0.69
Breast cancer (174)	15.8	13.7	16.8	18.0	..	15.3	10.9	15.1	1.7	2.5	0.17
Prostate cancer (185)	19.2	23.9	25.2	..	..	..	10.9	19.8	2.3	6.5	0.33
Diabetes Mellitus (250)	17.0	19.8	24.9	18.0	63.8	19.1	10.5	18.2	2.4	4.7	0.26
Inflammatory disease of the eye (360 +)	6.3	10.9	15.4	13.6	..	7.2	4.1	9.6	3.8	4.4	0.46
Otitis (380-382)	3.9	8.7	11.8	10.8	..	6.3	2.5	7.3	4.7	3.7	0.51
Rheumatic fever (390-398)	12.5	16.9	21.0	17.8	45.2	14.8	7.2	15.0	2.9	4.8	0.32
Hypertension (401-405)	12.7	16.2	23.4	15.7	75.8	17.1	7.0	15.4	3.3	5.4	0.35
Pneumonia (480-486)	12.4	16.8	28.9	16.8	19.3	46.1	8.3	21.6	5.6	13.9	0.64
Bronchitis (490-491)	9.1	16.9	21.3	..	..	12.4	6.2	13.2	3.4	6.0	0.46
Asthma (493)	6.3	16.9	21.3	11.3	44.1	12.4	6.0	12.4	3.6	6.0	0.48
Appendicitis (540-543)	6.0	9.4	11.2	9.2	10.1	6.6	5.4	8.0	2.1	2.3	0.29
Cholecystitis (574)	10.5	19.6	23.3	18.7	..	11.7	9.3	15.5	2.5	5.8	0.37
Nephritis (580-584)	13.2	10.5	17.2	19.1	..	..	10.6	14.1	1.8	3.9	0.28
Infections of skin (680-686)	7.3	10.8	16.2	11.3	..	13.2	7.3	11.0	2.2	3.4	0.31
Other diseases of tissue (690-698)	12.8	15.3	21.8	11.3	..	13.2	7.3	13.6	3.0	4.8	0.35
Osteoarthritis (715)	20.9	23.5	28.4	13.9	..	29.6	10.8	21.2	2.7	7.6	0.36

Note: * Excludes Japan.

Source: Measuring Health Care 1960-1983, OECD, Paris, 1985, Table E.3.

the high and the low. Similarly, the coefficients of variation are quite large, varying from 0.23 for Neoplasms to 0.76 for Mental Disorders.

Part of this variability in ALOS may be due to the aggregate level of the disease categories. Table 33 contains ALOS information for somatic hospitals for 1980 for these seven countries for 17 detailed ICD-subcategories. As above, the Japanese data are excluded from the summary statistics. Surprisingly, there is about the same amount of variation in lengths of stay for the detailed diagnoses codes as there is for the more aggregate classification. As above, for certain diagnoses, such as Pulmonary Tuberculosis, Otitis and Pneumonia, there is substantial variation across countries as shown by coefficients of variation greater than 0.50. For others, such as Breast Cancer, Diabetes Mellitus, Appendicitis and Nephritis, there is much less variation as evinced by coefficients of variation of less than 0.30. Perhaps, as discussed above, this relates to "professional uncertainty" regarding treatment. It may also relate to differences in intensity of services during the stay. Unfortunately, in the absence of outcome measures, judgements about relative efficiency or effectiveness across countries cannot easily be made. For example, the United States has the shortest length of stay in virtually every category; yet, as shown above, its per admission costs are among the highest. Nevertheless, substantial variations in lengths of stay exist across countries, even holding diagnosis constant.

Ambulatory Care

Ambulatory care is the second largest component of (public) health spending in most OECD countries. It is composed principally of spending on ambulatory physicians' services and ambulatory care facilities. Spending on ambulatory care is a critical determinant of overall health spending, because of the physician's central decision-maker/gatekeeper role, the cost-effectiveness of preventive services, and the potential substitutability of costly institutional for less costly ambulatory care services.

Ambulatory care expenditures as a percentage of all public health expenditures have increased slightly, rising from 20.2 per cent in 1970 to 21.3 per cent in the early 1980s. The prices of ambulatory care services for all countries increased at the second highest rate (after institutional prices), and slightly exceeded overall inflation. With respect to individual countries, in the 1980s ambulatory care spending ranged from 6.1 per cent in New Zealand to 37.7 per cent in Belgium[9]. In 1970, such spending ranged from 5.0 in the Netherlands to 39.2 in Belgium. Finland, the Netherlands and Sweden had the largest annual growth, while New Zealand and Norway had the lowest. With regard to increases in price, Japan, Sweden and Switzerland had the smallest price increases and Greece, Finland, Portugal and Italy the largest.

These observed differences in ambulatory care expenditures are due to differences in definitions, differences in delivery system characteristics, and differences in the provision and use of physician services. For example, the national source statistics underlying these data often do not permit the inclusion of outpatient hospital services in the ambulatory care classification. Moreover, there is no consistent international data source on total physician expenditures, or such spending disaggregated by place of service. However, data are available on the numbers of physicians, use of outpatient physician services, fees for certain medical procedures, and physicians' incomes. These data are analysed in order to provide some general insights into differences in availability and use of physician services across OECD countries.

Table 34 contains data on the number of physicians per 1 000 population in 1960, 1970, and the early 1980s. There has been substantial growth in the physician-population ratios in all OECD countries. The OECD average number of physicians per (1 000) capita has increased from 1.1 in 1960 to 1.2 in 1970 to 1.9 in the early 1980s. Cross-country differences in physician-population ratios as evinced by the coefficient of variation have remained about the same, with a coefficient of variation of about 0.25 in all three periods. In percentage terms, the average OECD physician-population ratio increased at an average annual rate of 4.2 per cent for the entire 1960-1980s period, 2.0 per cent between 1960-1970, and 4.8 per cent between 1970-1980s. All countries experienced substantial growth in their physician-population ratios over this period, and in all but two, the bulk of the growth took place after 1970. Finland, Italy, Portugal and Sweden experienced the largest growth, while Austria, Ireland, Japan and the United States had the lowest.

Much of this growth took place as a result of deliberate government policies to increase the number of physicians from levels that were perceived as inadequate in the 1950s and 1960s. But in the context of the 1970s and 1980s, the expansion of medical school capacities as well as the high rates of return to individuals from medical education have resulted in overall surpluses of physicians and restrictions on medical school enrolments in most OECD countries, although there continue to be shortages of physicians in certain specialties and geographic areas. However, reducing an increase in this surplus is difficult given the size of the stock relative to the flow, the long gestation period (e.g. the large number already in the training pipeline, irrespective of reductions in first-year placements), and the continued excess demand for medical education given the current expected returns (financial and professional) in most countries.

In addition to these factors, there are important consequences for health systems' performance from the number, growth and mix of specialists. The extent to which specialists, as opposed to generalists, provide care, the types of care they provide, the education and credentialling processes for specialists, and referral

Table 34

PHYSICIANS PER (1 000) CAPITA, 1960, 1970, 1980s

	Physicians per 1 000 population			Annual percentage growth		
	1960	1970	1980s	1960-70	1970-1980s	1960-1980s
Australia	1.1 (61)	1.3 (71)	1.9 (81)	1.8	4.6	3.6
Austria	1.4	1.4	1.7 (83)	0	1.6	0.9
Belgium	1.2	1.6	2.6 (81)	3.3	5.7	5.6
Canada	1.2 (61)	1.5	1.9 (82)	2.8	2.2	2.8
Denmark	1.3 (62)	1.5	2.4 (82)	1.9	5.0	4.2
Finland	0.6	1.0	2.2 (83)	6.7	9.2	11.6
France	1.0	1.3	2.2 (83)	3.0	5.3	5.2
Germany	1.4	1.6	2.4 (82)	1.4	4.2	3.2
Greece	1.3	1.6	2.5 (81)	2.3	5.1	4.4
Iceland	1.2	1.4	2.2 (81)	1.7	5.2	4.0
Ireland	1.0 (61)	1.2 (71)	1.2 (75)	2.0	0	1.4
Italy	0.5	0.7	1.3 (83)	4.0	13.8	7.0
Japan	1.0	1.1	1.4 (82)	1.0	2.3	1.8
Luxembourg	1.0	1.1	1.7 (83)	1.0	4.2	3.0
Netherlands	1.1	1.2	2.1 (83)	0.9	5.8	4.0
New Zealand	1.1	1.1 (71)	1.7 (83)	0	4.5	2.4
Norway	1.2	1.4	2.0 (81)	1.7	3.9	3.2
Portugal	0.8	0.9	2.1 (81)	1.3	2.0	7.7
Spain	1.2	1.3	2.6 (81)	0.8	9.1	5.6
Sweden	1.0	1.3	2.4 (83)	3.0	6.5	6.0
Switzerland*	1.0	1.1	1.6 (81)	1.0	4.1	2.9
Turkey	0.3	0.4	0.6 (81)	3.3	4.5	4.8
United Kingdom	-	1.0 (71)	1.3 (81)	-	3.0	-
United States	1.4	1.6	1.9 (81)	1.4	1.7	1.7
Average **	1.1	1.2	1.9	2.0	4.8	4.2
High - Low**	1.1	1.2	2.0	6.7	13.8	10.7
Standard Deviation**	0.3	0.3	0.5	1.5	2.9	2.4

Notes: * Data do not include full-time salaried physicians employed in hospitals. If these are included the ratio is 1.4 for 1970 and 2.5 for 1981. See Health Service Consultants, Eurocare, Basle, 1984.
** Excludes the United Kingdom.

Source: Measuring Health Care 1960-1983, OECD, Paris, 1985, Tables D.6 and H.1.

patterns among generalists and specialists all have important consequences for access, cost, quality and outcomes[10]. While such an analysis is beyond the scope of this report, the importance of these factors must be considered in interpreting the results below.

Increases in the supply of physicians could have either positive or negative effects on the fees paid and quantities of services (physician and others) provided, depending on whether physicians' behavioural responses to system reimbursement and coverage features result in competitive market solutions or supply-induced demand[11]. Obviously, the expenditure effects of increased physician supply will depend heavily on the way physicians are reimbursed, the manner in which other services (lab tests, pharmaceuticals, hospitals, etc.) are reimbursed, volume controls, and the open- or closed-endedness of the payment system. To theoretically test the behavioural hypotheses outlined above, detailed micro data and systems information, which are at present not readily accessible, would be needed. However, in order to provide some information on the general direction of these relationships, trends in physician outpatient consultations and the relationship between physician-population ratios and hospital use are analysed.

As shown in Table 35, outpatient physician consultations per capita increased from an OECD average (10 countries) of 5.0 in 1970 to 6.1 in the early 1980s, an average annual increase of 3.4 per cent. Over the same

Table 35

OUTPATIENT PHYSICIAN CONSULTATIONS, 1970, 1980s

Country	1970	1980s	Average annual percentage change
Australia	4.4	6.4 (81)	4.1
Austria	10.7	-	-
Belgium	-	7.1 (81)	-
Canada	-	5.5 (81)	-
Denmark	-	8.4 (82)	-
Finland	2.4	3.4 (83)	3.2
France	3.2	4.7 (83)	3.6
Greece	5.2	5.3 (82)	0.2
Iceland	-	4.9 (81)	-
Ireland	-	6.0 (82)	-
Italy	6.3	8.3 (81)	2.9
Japan	13.9	14.2 (78)	0.3
Netherlands	-	3.2 (80)	-
New Zealand	-	3.8 (81)	-
Norway	-	4.5 (83)	-
Portugal	1.5	3.8 (82)	12.8
Spain	2.6	4.7 (80)	8.1
Sweden	-	2.7 (83)	-
Switzerland	6.3	5.6 (82)	-0.9
Turkey	-	1.2 (81)	-
United Kingdom	-	4.2 (81)	-
United States	4.6	4.6 (81)	0
Mean*	5.0	6.1	3.4
High - Low*	12.4	10.8	13.7
Standard Deviation*	3.5	3.2	-
Mean - All Countries	5.6	5.4	4.2

Note: * For the 10 countries with data for both time periods.
Source: Measuring Health Care 1960-1983, OECD, Paris, 1985, Table D.2.

period the OECD physician to population ratio for these 10 countries increased by 5.8 per cent per year. In addition, for the early 1980s the cross-country correlation between number of outpatient consultations and physicians per capita is only -0.06 and is not statistically significant. These results, the relatively small increase in consultations relative to physicians and the low correlation are not surprising, since the physician consultation figures are only for outpatient consultations, while the physician-population ratios apply to all physicians.

To test the sensitivity of the various hospital use measures to physician availability, hospital days per capita, admission rates, average lengths of stay, and occupancy rates are each correlated with physicians per capita. The simple correlation coefficients are 0.07, 0.07, -0.22 and -0.01, respectively, and in no cases are the correlations statistically significant. While these results suggest that there is no cross-country relationship between physician supply and hospital use, these findings must be interpreted carefully[12]. First, the hospital data are not strictly comparable. Second, the physician statistics refer to all physicians, not only those with significant impacts on hospital use. To draw definitive conclusions more comparable data (e.g. short-term acute care hospitals), more detailed data (e.g. specialty, location of practice, and status with regard to admitting privileges of physicians) and information on reimbursement procedures for hospitals and physicians would be needed.

Fees paid for physician and other medical services can also significantly affect overall health spending and use of specific services. There are no internationally comparable detailed measures of the absolute or relative price levels of physician services for the OECD countries, although the OECD and the EEC are currently in the process of collecting such information in their updating of PPPs. However, some information on the absolute price levels of certain medical services are collected for a number of European countries by the *Association Internationale de la Mutualité* (AIM), a Geneva-based organisation of European mutual insurance organisations. In addition, fee data for Japan, Australia, and the United States Medicare programme were obtained from the Japanese Ministry of Health and Welfare, the Australian Commonwealth Department of Health, and the United States Department of Health and Human Services.

Table 36 contains the fees in local currencies and PPP-adjusted US dollars for 18 medical, surgical, laboratory, radiology, and dental procedures for Belgium, Germany, France, Luxembourg, the Netherlands, Denmark, Switzerland, Japan and the United States. The Australian data are not included here, although they are used in the relative fee analysis below, because they are for 1985-86 and appropriate PPP deflators were not available. These figures must be interpreted with caution, since procedures may not be defined exactly the same across countries and fees may vary by specialty of the physician or place of service (e.g. lab or physician's office). Where fees vary within a country, the maximum fee levels are chosen for inclusion in the table. In addition, since the data sources for Japan and the

Table 36

MEDICAL SERVICE FEES, 1984
(In local currency and US$ at PPPs)

	Belgium		Germany		France		Luxembourg		Netherlands		Denmark		Switzerland		European mean	European high/low	United States	Japan	
	BF	$	DM	$	FF	$	FL	$	Fl	$	K	$	SF	$	$		$	Y	$
1. GP home visit	430	12	29	14	81	13	680	18	--	--	89	11	52	24	15	2.2	31	2000	10
2. First consultation of internal medicine with major examination	659	18	21	10	95	15	1135	31	52	22	337	41	73	34	25	4.1	72	1350	7
3. Normal delivery by GP	5084	139	97	45	950	154	4055	109	604	258	446	54	449	207	138	5.7	--	--	--
4. Cholecystectomy	8317	227	293	136	920	149	7385	199	328	140	--	--	930	429	213	3.2	1754	80000	394
5. Total hysterectomy	8911	243	325	151	1150	187	8025	216	423	181	--	--	940	433	235	2.9	1754	61000	300
6. Appendectomy	4752	130	174	81	575	93	3805	103	188	80	--	--	560	258	124	3.2	1135	37500	185
7. Examination of urine	83	2	--	--	119	19	111	3	--	--	22	3	14	6	7	9.5	5	2450	12
8. Prothrombin time test	131	4	--	--	26	4	111	3	--	--	44	5	27	12	6	4.0	7	400	2
9. Total cholesterol dosage	136	4	--	--	17	3	134	4	--	--	68	8	42	19	8	6.3	5	600	3
10. Thorax radiography: 1. incidence	664	18	53	25	122	20	595	16	22	9	411	50	125	57	28	6.3	41	--	--
11. Colon radiography	3318	91	95	44	446	72	1355	37	58	25	454	55	397	183	72	7.3	155	--	--
12. Radiography of lombasacral column	1611	44	90	42	180	29	360	10	31	13	363	44	270	124	44	12.4	93	--	--
13. Electroencephalogram	2043	56	69	32	805	131	1055	28	86	37	219	26	245	113	60	4.3	125	5000	25
14. Electrocardiogram	530	14	30	14	92	15	525	14	--	--	88	11	84	39	18	3.5	45	1500	7
15. Bronchoscopy	1792	49	70	33	345	56	2425	65	153	65	398	48	212	97	59	2.9	413	3200	16
16. Rectosigmoidoscopy	754	21	106	49	115	19	850	23	117	50	398	48	235	108	45	5.7	72	900	4
17. Extraction of one lower molar	298	8	16	7	92	15	295	8	11	5	104	13	18	8	9	3.0	--	2400	12
18. Filling: one face	529	14	26	12	74	12	495	13	19	8	--	--	--	--	12	1.8	--	--	--

Notes: -- Data generally refer to 1984; however the data for the Netherlands, depending on the procedure, refer to 1981, 1982, 1983 or 1984. See sources below.

-- Where a choice among plans or a range of fees is presented, the maximum fee is chosen (e.g. the electroencephalogram fee for France). In the case of Switzerland, the differences between minimum and maximum fees are on the order of 2:1. The U.S. data are for Kings County (Manhattan), New York, the highest fee county in the United States, where fees are almost double the U.S. average.

-- Additional mileage charges for (GP) home visits are paid in Luxembourg, Denmark and Japan.

-- Fees may refer to different specialties; procedure definitions may not be exactly comparable; and there may be some non-comparability in terms of technical (e.g. lab) and professional (physician interpretation) components of various procedures.

Sources: Financing and Delivering Health Care: A Comparative Analysis of OECD Countries, OECD, Paris, 1987.

United States are different from the single European data source, the possibility of procedure definitional differences is compounded, and hence Japan and the United States are not included in the summary statistics.

Not surprisingly, there is a wide variation in PPP-adjusted fees across the nine countries. Even within Europe, there are fourfold or more differences in fees for more than half of the 18 procedures. Fees in Japan for physician visits and certain diagnostic and laboratory tests are below the European averages, but fees for surgical procedures are above the European average fees. The United States fees exceed the European averages in all but two cases, and five to sevenfold differences are found for certain surgical procedures. While these results should be interpreted with caution due to possible differences in the content of services, use of maximum as opposed to average fees in Switzerland and the United States, questions about whether the procedures chosen for individual countries are representative of overall fee structures, and differences in price levels within countries which are only roughly accounted for through the use of GDP PPPs, there do appear to be large absolute fee differentials across countries. Nevertheless, of more importance from a resource allocation perspective is the relative fee structure within countries.

In order to see if relative fee structures are similar across countries, the fees in each country were divided by the fee for an internist's consultation (procedure 2), yielding a relative value scale for each country[13]. Then each country's relative value scale was correlated against the relative value scales of all other countries for all common procedures for which fee data were available, using both Pearson (product movement) and Spearman (rank order) correlation techniques. The Pearson correlations measure the relationships among the magnitudes of the relative fees in each country, while the Spearman correlations provide only a measure of the rank ordering of the relative fees. The resulting correlation matrices are presented in Table 37.

Relative fee distributions in terms of their actual magnitudes are highly interrelated (e.g. correlation of 0.94 or more) among Australia, Belgium, Germany, Japan, Switzerland and the United States. In other words the prices of different medical procedures relative to the price of a first internal medicine visit are remarkably similar. Perhaps this is due to the historical influence of the German medical system on the Belgian, Swiss and Japanese systems, coupled with the influences of the American medical system on the Australian, Japanese and German systems following the Second World War. In any event the correlations are consistently high among all these countries. The Dutch system is highly correlated (0.95) with the United States system but not as much with the others, and the relative fees in Luxembourg are highly correlated (0.96) with those in Japan. Relative fees in France, and to a lesser extent Denmark, are not highly correlated with those in other countries. These relationships tend to be confirmed by the Spearman correlations, which indicate more consistency in terms of the rank ordering of relative fees, but, of course, do not take into account their relative magnitudes.

Given the caveats cited above, the preceding analysis cannot be regarded as definitive. Nevertheless, it does suggest that there are some strong basic similarities in relative medical prices across several countries. These would appear to relate to the historical antecedents of the various systems as well as cross-national flows of medical technology and practice. Unfortunately, on the basis of this analysis, general prognostications about

Table 37

CORRELATIONS OF 1984 RELATIVE FEES

	Belgium	Germany	France	Luxembourg	Netherlands	Denmark	Switzerland	United States	Japan	Australia (85)
					(Pearson Correlations)					
Belgium		0.94	0.60	0.72	0.78	0.67	0.99	0.97	0.97	0.98
Germany	0.88		0.59	0.59	0.62	0.75	0.98	0.96	0.95	0.97
France	0.71	0.71		0.38	0.52	0.66	0.63	0.50	0.62	0.62
Luxembourg	0.82	0.71	0.65		0.37	0.52	0.71	0.55	0.96	0.60
Netherlands	0.91	0.84	0.55	0.78		0.39	0.69	0.95	0.89	0.75
Denmark	0.86	0.95	0.77	0.82	0.43		0.80	0.56	0.19	0.57
Switzerland	0.97	0.93	0.72	0.84	0.96	0.83		0.95	0.96	0.97
United States	0.98	0.78	0.60	0.87	0.84	0.74	0.92		0.98	0.97
Japan	0.73	0.64	0.64	0.77	0.76	0.47	0.64	0.83		0.95
Australia (85)	0.94	0.96	0.84	0.87	0.90	0.80	0.94	0.89	0.69	
					(Spearman Correlations)					

Sources: Table 36.
  Data for Australia are from Medical Benefits Schedule Book, Commonwealth Department of Health, Canberra, 1986. Fees are for 1st July, 1985 for New South Wales. Procedure numbers and fees in $Aus. corresponding to procedures 1-16, respectively, in Table 36 are: 15 - $22.50, 5 - $15.60, 200 - $225, 3798 - $405, 6533 - $500, 4080 - $225, 1504 - $11.40, 1234 - $11.40, 1301 - $17.20, 2627 - $36.50, 2711 - $90, 2601 - $63, 803 - $75, 908 - $26.50, 5605 - $97, 4367 - $102.

which procedures are under- or over-valued relative to others and the concomitant resource allocation effects of such relative valuations cannot be made. For example, there is a major debate in the United States about the over-valuation of surgical and diagnostic procedures relative to "cognitive" care. To the extent that the United States fee structure reflects such price distortions, it would appear that the Australian, Belgian, Swiss, Japanese and German relative fee structures also reflect the same distortions. On the other hand, nothing can be said about the presence or absence of these distortions in the other four countries. Furthermore, the resource allocation effects will also depend on hospital admission policies, the methods used to reimburse physicians, laboratories and hospitals, availability of physicians and hospital beds, mix of public and private programmes, etc.

Much of the debate on physician cost containment and reimbursement reform is predicated on the perceived privileged income position of physicians. While economists cannot readily answer the question of whether specific physician income levels are too high (or too low), excess demand for medical school placements and studies in individual countries indicate that the rates of return to medical education generally exceed those of other comparable occupations[14]. This excess demand for medical education exacerbates the problem of physician surpluses in many countries[15].

Table 38 displays the incomes of physicians in 16 OECD countries, both as a ratio to average employee compensation and in absolute US$ using GDP PPPs for 1970 and 1981. These data must be interpreted with caution, since they may mask significant differences in employment relationships of the physicians surveyed, hours worked and specialty-mix. On average, physician incomes are 2.8 times that of the average employee, ranging from 1.1 in Italy to 5.1 in the United States. The ratios are the highest in the United States, Japan and Germany, and the lowest in Italy, Ireland and Norway. However, the ratios have fallen since 1970, when the OECD average ratio was 3.5. The studies cited in note 14 also indicate that the rates of return have fallen. This may reflect increased government cost containment and/or increased competition engendered by substantial growth in the supply of physicians.

In terms of absolute income levels, in 1981, physician incomes for the 16 OECD countries averaged $46 800, ranging from $18 200 in Ireland to $93 000 in the United States. Physicians in the United States, Switzerland, Germany, Canada and Japan had the highest incomes, while those in Ireland, Italy and Finland had the lowest. In 1970 the rankings were quite similar.

While these data are of interest in describing the income positions of physicians, and are sometimes used as a political rationale for imposing physician cost containment measures, the importance of the physician's central decision-making role must be kept in mind. While physicians themselves account for less than 10 per cent of all people employed in the health sector

Table 38

PHYSICIAN INCOMES, 1970, 1981

	Relative to average employee income		Absolute amount (US$ GDP PPPs)	
	1970	1981	1970	1981
Australia	4.3	2.5	$25 600	$41 500
Belgium	-	1.8	-	35 500
Canada	5.1	4.1	37 800	72 700
Denmark	-	2.8 (80)	-	38 400 (80)
Finland	3.7	1.8	16 200	24 200
France	4.8	3.3 (79)	26 600	46 800 (79)
Germany	6.4 (71)	4.9 (80)	40 800 (71)	76 300 (80)
Ireland	1.5	1.2	14 200	18 200
Italy	1.4	1.1	8 600	19 600
Japan	-	4.7	-	68 200
New Zealand	-	2.5	21 400	33 300
Norway	2.4 (71)	1.7	16 800 (71)	28 500
Sweden	3.7	2.1	25 500	35 300
Switzerland	-	-	34 500	84 200
United Kingdom	-	2.4	-	32 300
United States	5.4	5.1	41 800	93 000
Average	3.5	2.8	25 800	46 800
High/Low	3.9	4.6	4.9	5.1
Standard deviation	1.7	1.3	11 000	24 100

Sources: Measuring Health Care 1960-1983, OECD, Paris, 1985, Tables B.6.D. and H.5.
National Accounts Main Aggregate, Volume 1, OECD, Paris, 1986.
Data for Japan are revised Secretariat estimates based on differential compensation weights for salaried physicians and physician owners of clinics and hospitals.

and receive on the order of less than 25 per cent of all health expenditures, their decisions affect 70-80 per cent of all spending[16]. Reducing physician expenditures by 10 per cent will only save 2 per cent of all spending. If physicians react to such measures by substituting hospital, pharmaceutical, or other services, overall spending may well increase. The facetious proposal to pay surgeons not to operate is indeed predicated on this important precept of the physician as the central decision-maker. In addition, it is interesting to note that of the six physician-associated cost-increasing factors identified by Schroeder[17]

i)   a high concentration of physicians and of specialists,

ii) fee-for-service payment of specialists and generalists,

iii) patient self-referral directly to specialists,

iv) physicians permitted to practice a specialty independent of the specialty certification process,

v)   a high dependence on specialists for primary care, and

vi) broad national health insurance –

the countries with high physician incomes generally tend to meet more of these criteria than those with low physician incomes.

Pharmaceuticals

Pharmaceutical expenditures are the third largest component of public health expenditures. As a percentage of all public health expenditures, pharmaceutical expenditures decreased from an OECD average of 12.4 per cent of total spending in 1970 to 9.9 per cent in the 1980s. Pharmaceutical prices increased at a 12.6 per cent annual rate, the slowest growing health care price component. Pharmaceutical prices increased less rapidly than overall consumer prices and the GDP deflator[18]. With regard to individual countries, public pharmaceutical expenditures in 1970 ranged from less than one per cent of all public spending in Canada to 36.8 per cent in Spain. By the 1980s public spending on pharmaceuticals ranged from 1.5 per cent in the United States to over 20 per cent in Portugal. Canada and Ireland had the highest growth in pharmaceutical spending, while Australia and Spain had the lowest.

Table 39 displays per capita pharmaceutical expenditures and consumption for the OECD countries for 1970 and the 1980s. These data must be interpreted with caution, since pharmaceuticals consumed in hospitals are generally reported as hospital expenditures, and outpatient pharmaceutical expenditures and consumption may be understated[19]. Per capita pharmaceutical expenditures in GDP PPPs increased from a 1970 OECD average of $35 to $99 in the early 1980s. In the early 1980s per capita expenditures varied from $42 in Denmark to $194 in Germany. Pharmaceutical consumption, prescriptions per person (measured in numbers of prescriptions not dosage units), has increased from an OECD average of 9.9 prescriptions in the early 1970s to 10.4 in the early 1980s. The countries with the highest consumption in terms of numbers of prescriptions are France and Italy, while the lowest consumption

is in the United States and Sweden. However, there does not appear to be a strong relationship between expenditures per capita and prescriptions per capita as evinced by a correlation (not statistically significant) of 0.36. This result (as well as a considerably amount of direct evidence based on surveys) would suggest that internal pricing policies vary widely among countries. Furthermore, as far as consumption of pharmaceuticals is concerned, although it would be expected, *ceteris paribus*, that the more physicians and pharmacists per capita, the greater the use of pharmaceuticals, the cross-country data indicate no significant relationships between expenditures or consumption with physicians or pharmacists per capita (no correlation exceeded 0.3 in absolute magnitude).

Other Health Expenditures

This category covers all other medical services including therapeutic appliances, biomedical research, etc. Since it is calculated as a residual (e.g. institutional, ambulatory and pharmaceutical expenditures are subtracted from the total), it also could be picking up expenditures associated with classification errors or differences in service definitions. Public expenditures on other health services accounted for an OECD average of 18.2 per cent of all spending in 1970 and 16.5 per cent in the 1980s.

Table 39

PHARMACEUTICAL EXPENDITURES PER CAPITA AND CONSUMPTION, 1970, 1980s

	1970		1980s		Annual percentage change	
	Expenditures per capita (US$, GDP PPPs)	Number of prescriptions per capita	Expenditures per capita (US$, GDP PPPs)	Number of prescriptions per capita	Expenditures per capita (US$, GDP PPPs)	Number of prescriptions per capita
Australia	49.2 (75)	7.2 (75)	78.7 (82)	7.5 (81)	8.6	0.7
Austria	10.9	16.3	46.0 (84)	14.9 (81)	23.0	-0.8
Belgium	53.7	"	127.8 (82)	9.9 (82)	11.5	"
Canada	36.0	-	101.6 (82)	"	15.2	"
Denmark	12.9	"	42.4 (83)	6.3 (83)	17.6	"
Finland	26.2	4.0	79.2 (83)	4.9 (82)	15.6	1.9
France	56.5	17.4	188.1 (84)	28.9 (81)	16.6	6.0
Germany	46.2	"	194.1 (82)	"	26.7	"
Greece	29.9	5.8	73.7 (82)	7.4 (82)	12.2	2.3
Iceland	-	"	"	4.8 (79)	"	"
Ireland	27.1	-	67.4 (81)	11.9 (81)	13.5	"
Italy	26.5	10.9	110.1 (83)	21.5 (77)	24.3	13.9
Japan	-	"	"	"	"	"
Luxembourg	45.7	11.3	138.5 (84)	12.4 (78)	14.5	1.2
Netherlands	17.5	9.1	104.3 (84)	"	35.4	"
New Zealand	-	6.8	"	8.5 (83)	"	1.9
Norway	14.9	"	50.1 (84)	5.6 (77)	16.9	"
Portugal	-	14.8	61.7 (81)	15.5 (81)	"	"
Spain	-	9.2	75.7 (80)	11.9 (83)	"	"
Sweden	42.7 (73)	"	104.2 (83)	4.6 (83)	14.4	"
Switzerland	53.6	"	134.8 (82)	"	12.6	"
Turkey	-	"	"	"	"	"
United Kingdom	"	5.5	"	6.8 (82)	"	"
United States	39.0	"	109.0 (84)	4.3 (77)	12.8	"
Mean	34.6	9.9	99.3	10.4	17.1	3.4
Range	45.6	13.4	151.7	24.6	26.8	14.7
Standard Deviation	15.2	4.4	43.3	6.5	6.7	4.7

Sources: Measuring Health Care 1960-83, OECD, Paris, 1985, Tables A.7 and D.3. Figures for 1984 are preliminary OECD Secretariat estimates.
National Accounts, Main Aggregates, Volume I, OECD, Paris, 1986.

Given the residual and aggregate nature of this category, it is difficult to discuss it in policy-relevant terms. However, to the extent that it includes therapeutic appliances and supplies such as cardiac pacemakers, infusion pumps, intraocular lenses, and parenteral and enteral nutrients, these items could have significant expenditure impacts in the future, as new therapeutic techniques coupled with changing disease patterns resulting from ageing populations put extensive demands on these services. Similarly, amounts spent on biomedical research could also have significant but less direct, although at this point unpredictable, impacts on future health expenditures.

NOTES AND REFERENCES

1. See discussions of these problems in *Measuring Health Care 1960-1983*, OECD, Paris, 1985; Brian Abel-Smith (ed.), *Eurocare*, Health Econ. Basle, Switzerland; and Robert A. Maxwell, *Health and Wealth: An International Study of Health Care Spending*, Lexington Books, Lexington, Massachusetts, 1981.

2. Robert A. Maxwell, *Health and Wealth: An International Study of Health Care Spending, Ibid.*

3. See Mark R. Chassan, *Variations in Hospital Length of Stay: Their Relationship to Health Outcomes*, Health Technology Case Study 24, United States Office of Technology Assessment, Washington, D.C., 1983.

4. Sizeable and unexplainable differences in costs per day and per admission were also found in a micro-costing study of hospitals in 5 OECD countries. See *The Cost of Hospitalisation Micro-economic Approach to the Problems Involved*, Social Policy Series No. 39, Commission of the European Communities, Brussels, 1979.

5. *Health United States 1985*, United States Department of Health and Human Services, National Center for Health Statistics, Hyattsville, Maryland, 1985, p. 144.

6. These and the other hospital use data should be interpreted with caution since definitions across countries are not strictly comparable. See *Measuring Health Care 1960-1983, op.cit.*, pp. 95-103.

7. M.I. Roemer, "Bed Supply and Hospital Utilisation: A Natural Experiment", *Hospitals*, November 1, 1961.

8. This statistic is sensitive to the countries included and indeed would be significant if a 0.15 instead of a 0.05 significance level was used. For example a statistically significant relationship was found using 1980 data for 15 countries. See George J. Schieber, "The Financing and Delivery of Health Care in OECD Countries: Past, Present, and Future", in *Health and Pension Policies Under Economic and Demographic Constraints*, OECD, Paris, 1987.

9. Excluding Turkey where there appear to be some data anomalies.

10. See Steven A. Schroeder, "Western European Responses to Physician Oversupply", *Journal of the American Medical Association*, Vol. 252, No. 3, July 21, 1984; and Jan Blanpain, Bjorn Lindgren and Simone Sandier, *Comparaisons Internationales des Systèmes de Santé*, Centre de Recherche, d'Etude et de Documentation en Economie de la Santé, Paris, 1985.

11. For a discussion of the supply-induced demand versus competitive market hypotheses of physician behaviour, see Uwe Reinhardt, "The Theory of Physician-Induced Demand Reflections After a Decade", *Journal of Health Economics*, Vol. 4, 1985.

12. Some studies conducted within individual countries have found significant direct relationships between physician supply and hospital use. See J.W. Hurst, *Financing Health Services in the United States, Canada, and Britain*, King Edward's Hospital Fund, London, 1985.

13. This procedure is not really necessary, since correlations are not affected by linear transformations of the variables. However, it is more directly comprehensible for health policy-makers who think in terms of relative value schedules.

14. See, for example, Rob Wilson, "Changing Pay Relativities For the Highly Qualified", *Review of the Economy and Employment*, Vol. 2, 1985/86, University of Warwick, Institute for Employment Research, Coventry 1986; J.P. Jarousse, "Une Mesure de la Rentabilité des Diplômes Entre 1969 et 1976", *Consommation*, No. 2, 1985/86; and Monica Noether, "The Growing Supply of Physicians: Has the Market Become More Competitive?", *Journal of Labor Economics*, Vol. 4, No. 4, 1986.

15. Steven A. Schroeder, "Western European Responses to Physician Oversupply", *op.cit.*

16. See Simone Sandier, "Access, Quality and Efficiency: Physicians, Pharmaceuticals, and Other Ambulatory Services", in *Health and Pension Policies Under Economic and Demographic Constraints, op.cit.*

17. See Steven A. Schroeder, "Western European Responses to Physician Oversupply", *op.cit.*, pp. 381-382.

18. Pharmaceutical price indices must be interpreted with caution given the rapid introduction of new as well as improved products.

19. See *Measuring Health Care 1960-1983*, OECD, Paris, 1985, p. 20.

Chapter 7

CROSS-COUNTRY DIFFERENCES IN HEALTH SPENDING

The previous discussion has focused on analysing trends in health care spending and service composition within individual countries. This section analyses the factors associated with differences and changes in health spending across countries. First, the simple relationship between per capita health expenditures and the share of health in GDP relative to per capita GDP are estimated. Second, statistical relationships are developed which associate per capita health spending and the share of health in GDP with various other economic, demographic and health delivery system characteristics for the 1970, 1976 and 1982 time periods. Third, changes in health expenditures are statistically related to changes in these same factors.

Relationship between Health Expenditures and GDP

The simple relationship between health spending (per capita and health-GDP shares) and per capita GDP is important, since it provides information on whether wealthier countries tend to spend more on health. This relationship can be specified in a variety of different functional forms. Since *a priori* theoretical considerations do not impose a specific functional form and since the results obtained below from linear and logarithmic formulations are the same, the discussion here is based on linear specifications. However, the results from the logarithmic formulations are displayed in the appropriate tables.

Chart 12 shows the relationship between per capita health expenditures and per capita GDP for 21 OECD countries for 1984. The data points clearly indicate an upward trend, countries with higher per capita GDPs have higher per capita health expenditures. The fitted trend line indicates a statistically significant relationship in which each $100 difference in per capita GDP is associated with a $10.50 difference in per capita health expenditures. In terms of percentage differences, the calculated elasticity of health spending relative to GDP of 1.4 indicates that a 10 per cent difference in per capita GDP is associated with a 14 per cent difference in per capita health spending. Furthermore, the statistical analysis indicates that variations in per capita GDP,

alone, account for 77 per cent of the variation in per capita health spending. These results are generally consistent with those found in other studies and, as shown below, for other time periods[1].

In addition to analysing absolute differences in health spending, it is also of interest to analyse the relationship between per capita GDP and the proportion of GDP devoted to health. Chart 13 displays the relationship between the health to GDP share and per capita GDP for the same 21 OECD countries for 1984. A positive statistically significant relationship is again found, indicating that countries with higher per capita GDPs spend a larger proportion of their GDP on health. An elasticity of 0.51 is observed, indicating that a 10 per cent difference in per capita GDP is associated with a 5.1 per cent difference in the share of GDP devoted to health. Variations in per capita GDP are associated with 34 per cent of the variation in GDP shares.

Effects of Other Economic and Demographic Factors on Cross-Country Differences in Health Expenditures

Other economic and demographic factors would be expected on *a priori* theoretical grounds to be associated with differences in health spending. Ideally, a theoretical economic model of the supply of and demand for health services would be specified, a series of equations expressing endogenous and exogenous interrelationships would be derived, and then the parameters of these relationships would be estimated. However, given the present unavailability of much of the relevant economic data as well as the difficulties in developing such a model, the approach followed here is simply to develop empirical relationships among health spending and supply and demand factors for which data are available and relationships can be posited on *a priori* theoretical grounds.

Thus, both per capita health spending and the share of GDP devoted to health are empirically related to countries' age structures, availability of doctors and hospitals, and the public shares of total health spending. Countries with larger percentages of their population aged 65 and over and/or higher physician and hospital

Chart 12

PER CAPITA HEALTH SPENDING, PER CAPITA GDP, 1984

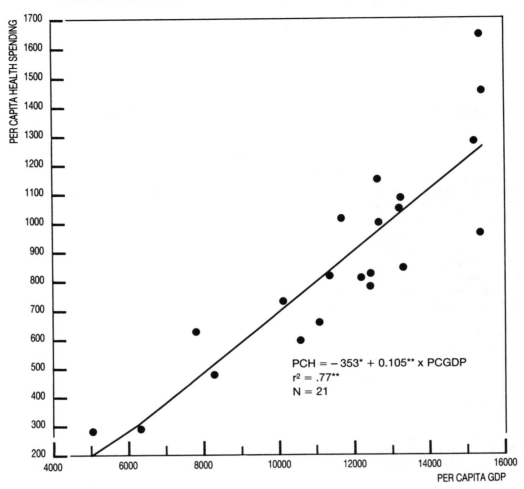

PCH = − 353* + 0.105** x PCGDP
r² = .77**
N = 21

Notes : PCH = Per capita total health spending in GDP PPPs.
PCGDP = Per capita GDP in GDP PPPs.
r² = Adjusted correlation coefficient squared.
N = Number of countries.
* = Statistically significant at the .05 level.
** = Statistically significant at the .01 level.
Excludes Luxembourg, Switzerland, and Turkey.
The equation for the logarithmic formulation is :
Log (PCH) = − 2.93** + 1.44** x Log (PCGDP)
r² = .87**
N = 21.

Source : Table 20.

bed to population ratios would be expected to have higher absolute and relative health expenditures, *ceteris paribus*. *A priori* expectations about the public share of total spending are less clear. To the extent that higher public shares are associated with higher eligibility ratios, fuller benefits and less cost-sharing, a higher public share would be expected to be associated with higher per capita spending and GDP shares. On the other hand, if most individuals have access to public programmes or subsidised private coverage, higher public penetration may be associated with better control over the health system and, hence, lower absolute and relative spending.

The analysis is performed on 1982 data, since the relevant information is available for 20 countries for which the same consistent data are also available for

Chart 13

HEALTH-GDP SHARE, PER CAPITA GDP, 1984

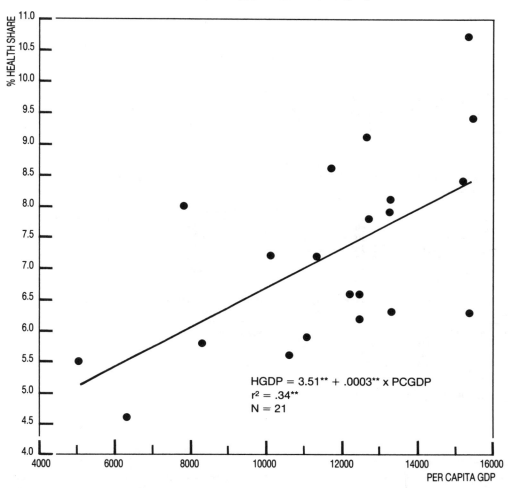

HGDP = 3.51** + .0003** x PCGDP
r² = .34**
N = 21

Notes : HGDP = Total health expenditures as a percent of GDP.
Same as Chart 12.
The equation for the logarithmic formulation is:
Log (HGDP) = − 0.91 + 0.43** x Log (PCGDP)
r² = .35**
N = 21.

Source : Table 20.

1970 and 1976, enabling the historical validity of the estimated structural relationships to be tested. Table 40 contains the estimated relationships between health spending (both per capita and GDP shares) and per capita GDP, public share, hospital beds per 1 000 capita, physicians per 1 000 capita, and per cent of population aged 65 and over. Inclusion of these other factors in the analysis adds little to the previous simple regression analysis for 1984. Per capita GDP is the only statistically significant factor (although the signs of the public share variable are consistently negative and would be statistically significant if a less rigorous

significance test was employed), and after controlling for the effects of differences in public share, hospital and physician availability, and percent of elderly population, the relationship between per capita GDP and health spending (both per capita and GDP share) is virtually the same as that found above for the simple relationship among the 21 countries for 1984.

In fact, the simple relationships between these factors and per capita health expenditures and health to GDP ratios are quite weak. Percentage of population aged 65 and over, physicians per 1 000 capita, hospital beds per 1 000 capita, and public share are each generally

Table 40

MULTIPLE REGRESSION ANALYSIS OF HEALTH EXPENDITURES
AND OTHER DEMOGRAPHIC AND ECONOMIC FACTORS, 1970, 1976, 1982

Year	Form	r^2	Constant	GDP per capita		Public share	Hospital beds per capita	Physicians per capita	Per cent population 65+
				Per Capita Health Expenditures					
1970	Linear	0.68**	-68.85	0.074**	[1.29]	-1.07	4.13	53.36	-2.36
	Log	0.70**	-1.80	1.28**		-0.38	0.22	0.14	0.01
1976	Linear	0.76**	-61.24	0.088**	[1.24]	-2.80	9.18	57.30	-1.66
	Log	0.75**	-1.27	1.15**		-0.41	0.24	0.19	0.01
1982	Linear	0.70**	55.66	0.106**	[1.39]	-4.87	-4.29	-22.54	6.73
	Log	0.72**	-1.84	1.33**		-0.34	-0.05	-0.03	0.06
Pooled	Linear	0.92**	36.35	0.089**	[1.24]	-3.17** [-0.47]	3.74	4.35	3.10
	Log	0.94**	-1.69**	1.27**		-0.36**	0.11	0.06	0.04
				Health-GDP Shares					
1970	Linear	0.16	3.69	0.0004	[0.29]	-0.03	0.13	1.34	-0.08
	Log	0.16	0.20	0.28		-0.35	0.24	0.15	-0.05
1976	Linear	0.24	5.76*	0.0002	[0.22]	-0.04	0.15	0.97	-0.03
	Log	0.23	0.77	0.14		-0.40	0.24	0.20	0.002
1982	Linear	0.13	7.60*	0.0002	[0.14]	-0.04	-0.03	-0.27	0.05
	Log	0.10	0.14	0.34		-0.34	-0.04	-0.03	0.06
Pooled	Linear	0.42**	6.43**	0.0002**	[0.25]	-0.04** [-0.39]	0.07	0.28	0.01
	Log	0.47**	0.31	0.27**		-0.35**	0.11	0.06	0.02

Notes: Based on 20 OECD countries, excluding Greece, Luxembourg, Portugal and Turkey.
    ** = statistically significant at the .01 level.
    * = statistically significant at the .05 level.
    r^2 = adjusted multiple correlation coefficient squared.
    [ ] = calculated elasticity.

Source: Measuring Health Care 1960-1983, OECD, Paris, 1985.

associated with less than 15 per cent of the variation (simple correlation coefficient squared) in per capita health spending and health to GDP ratios. In fact none of these correlations is statistically significant.

Furthermore, these factors are generally not associated with per capita GDP either. Age structure, physicians, hospital beds and public share are also each generally associated with less than 15 per cent of the variation in per capita GDP. As above, none of these correlations are statistically significant.

These results may appear counter-intuitive on *a priori* grounds, but an analysis of the basic data provides some answers. With respect to hospital bed and physician-population ratios, the data indicate that the countries with the highest (lowest) absolute and relative spending do not tend to have the highest (lowest) ratios. In fact, as indicated by the correlation analysis, there does not appear to be any consistent relationship. Countries with relatively low health spending such as Greece, Spain and Japan have high physician and/or hospital bed to population ratios. There are also undoubtedly definitional differences as well as qualitative differences in these resource measures. Definitional problems aside,

there are undoubtedly strong differences in intensity of services across countries that are unrelated to numbers of hospital beds and doctors, but which are likely to be significant determinants of spending differences.

Similar comments apply to the absence of any age-related effects. The United States, Canada and the Netherlands, high expenditure countries, tend to have relatively small proportions of their population over 65, while lower expenditure countries such as Austria, Belgium and Italy tend to have relatively larger older populations.

To test the validity of these relationships over time, the cross-country analysis was repeated for 1970 and 1976. The results indicate the same basic structural relationships for the three time periods. Per capita GDP is consistently the only statistically significant factor associated with differences in per capita health spending across countries. On the other hand, the relationship between per capita GDP and the share of health in GDP is not statistically significant, although the coefficients are consistent in terms of sign and magnitude and would be significant if a less rigorous statistical test was used, or if other variables were dropped from the analysis.

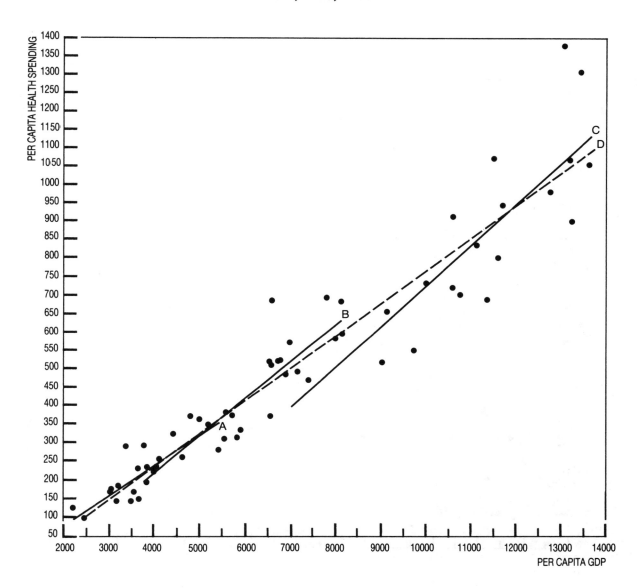

Chart 14

**PER CAPITA HEALTH SPENDING, PER CAPITA GDP,
1970, 1976, 1982**

Notes : PCH = Per capita health expenditure in GDP PPPs.
PCGDP = Per capita GDP in GDP PPPs.
N = Number of observations.
** = Statistically significant at .01 level.
* = Statistically significant at .05 level.
r^2 = Adjusted correlation coefficient squared.
(A) : (1970) PCH = − 85.5 + .08** x PCGDP
N = 20. r^2 = .67**
(B) : (1976) PCH = − 187.4 + .10** x PCGDP
N = 20. r^2 = .71**
(C) : (1982) PCH = − 377.9 + .11** x PCGDP
N = 20. r^2 = .70**
(D) : (1970, 76, 82) PCH = − 121.3** + .09** x PCGDP
N = 60. r^2 = .91**
Equations are simple regressions and hence coefficients differ slightly from the multiple regressions in
Table 40.

Source : Same as Table 40.

Chart 15

HEALTH-GDP SHARE, PER CAPITA GDP, 1970, 1976, 1982

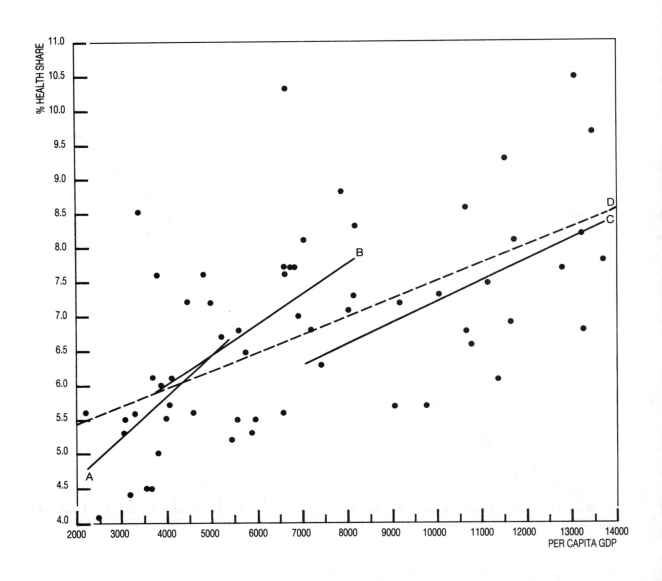

Notes : See Chart 14.
HGDP = Total health expenditures as a percent of GDP.
(A) : (1970) HGDP = 3.4* + .0006 x PCGDP
N = 20.   r² = .11
(B) : (1976) HGDP = 4.3* + .0004 x PCGDP
N = 20.   r² = .12
(C) : (1982) HGDP = 4.1* + .0003* x PCGDP
N = 20.   r² = .17*
(D) : (1970, 76, 82) HGDP = 4.9 ** + .0003** x PCGDP
N = 60.   r² = .34**

Source : Same as Table 40.

While the observed and calculated elasticities of per capita GDP do differ slightly depending on the years and mathematical formulation, the basic story is unchanged. Furthermore, statistical analyses of the estimated relationships for each pair of time periods indicate that there are no differences in the structural relationships among the three time periods.

Given this similarity of structural relationships, the data for each of the three time periods are pooled and the relationships between health expenditures and its associated factors are re-estimated. The results obtained from the pooled data are somewhat stronger, as expected, given the increased number of observations. In addition, the structural relationships are the same with one exception, the public share variable is statistically significant. For the per capita health expenditure analysis, the GDP elasticity is 1.24, while the public share elasticity is –0.47. No other factors are statistically significant. However, variations in all these factors account for 92 per cent of the variation in per capita health expenditures.

Similar results are found for the pooled data for the health-GDP ratio. Both per capita GDP and the public share are statistically significantly related, while other factors are not. The GDP elasticity is 0.25, and the public share elasticity is –0.39. Variations in the independent factors account for 42 per cent of the variation in health GDP shares.

The similarity of the structural relationships for the three time periods is shown in Charts 14 and 15, which display the data points and the simple trend lines for each time period and the trend line for the three time periods combined for per capita health expenditures and the health-GDP ratio relative to per capita GDP.

Cross-Country Analysis of Changes in Health Expenditures

It is also of interest to see if changes in per capita health expenditures and health-GDP shares are associated with changes in these demographic and health systems' characteristics. Changes in health expenditures between 1970 and 1976, 1976 and 1982, and 1970 and 1982 are statistically related to changes in per capita GDP, public share, hospital- and physician-population ratios and percent of population aged 65 and over for the same respective time periods. The results are displayed in Table 41. These new results concerning changes in health expenditures relative to changes in various explanatory factors are quite consistent with the previous ones: per capita GDP appears as the dominant explanatory factor with the public share factor significant in certain cases.

With regard to changes in per capita health expenditures, for all three time periods, the change in per capita GDP is consistently statistically significant and the major explanatory factor. The respective elasticities are 1.10, 1.24 and 1.15. Changes in the public share are statistically significantly related to changes in per capita health expenditures only for the 1976 to 1982 period, and the relationship is negative with an elasticity of – 0.06. Changes in hospital beds and physicians per capita and changes in the percent of population 65 and

Table 41

MULTIPLE REGRESSION ANALYSIS OF CHANGES IN HEALTH SPENDING
AND CHANGES IN OTHER DEMOGRAPHIC AND ECONOMIC FACTORS

Period	Dependent variable	r^2	Constant	GDP per capita	Public share	Hospital beds per capita	Physicians per capita	Per cent population 65+
1970-76	Per capita health expenditure	0.47*	-30.91	0.100** [1.10]	1.11	-1.47	68.92	-19.11
1976-82	Per capita health expenditure	0.36*	-50.32	0.103** [1.24]	-9.46* [-0.06]	-20.07	24.64	-52.62
1970-82	Per capita health expenditure	0.57**	-248.89	0.125** [1.15]	-6.88	-25.43	96.21	-44.46
1970-76	Health GDP share	-0.13	2.32**	-0.0003	0.004	0.08	0.78	-0.30
1976-82	Health GDP share	0.36*	1.25	-0.0001	-0.11** [-0.51]	-0.11	0.50	-0.39
1970-82	Health GDP share	0.44*	2.20	0.00003	-0.09** [-0.29]	-0.15	1.10	-0.50* [-0.46]

Notes: Based on 20 OECD countries excluding Greece, Luxembourg, Portugal and Turkey.
All multiple regressions are based on changes in the linear (non-log) variables.
** = statistically significant at the .01 level.
 * = statistically significant at the .05 level.
[ ] = calculated elasticity.

Source: Measuring Health Care 1960-1983, OECD, Paris, 1985.

over are not related statistically to changes in per capita health spending. All the explanatory factors accounted for 47 per cent of the variation in changes in per capita health spending between 1970-76, 36 per cent between 1976-82, and 57 per cent between 1970-82[2].

The estimated relationships between health-GDP shares and the explanatory factors are even weaker. The 1970-76 relationship is not statistically significant, while the other two time periods are significant at a 0.05, not 0.01, level. Changes in per capita GDP are not statistically significantly associated with changes in health to GDP ratios. However, the public share variables are statistically significantly related in both the 1976-82 and 1970-82 time periods. The calculated elasticities are – 0.51 and – 0.29, respectively. None of the other variables is statistically significant for any of the time periods except the age factor in the 1970-82 period. The percent of variation of changes in shares accounted for by the analysis is 36 per cent for 1976-82 and 44 per cent for 1970-82.

In summary, the analysis above indicates that both currently and historically, countries with higher per capita GDPs spend more on health services, and that higher public shares tend to be related with lower expenditures. Similarly, changes in per capita health expenditures also appear to be directly related to changes in GDP, while changes in health-GDP shares tend to be inversely related to changes in the public share.

Several caveats are, however, in order. The above analysis is purely statistical and is not based on a formal behavioural model of the medical care market. As such, causality cannot be attributed. Second, it is clear that the complex interrelationships among decision-makers, financing entities, reimbursement arrangements, and institutional structures are difficult both to define and measure. Crude macro measures of resource availability, such as physician or hospital bed to population ratios, do not adequately measure inputs, since they do not account for intensity of service. Measures of public penetration mask large differences in characteristics of public systems, such as those between a highly governmentally controlled British system relative to a more consensus-oriented German social insurance system. Moreover, data on critical expenditure determinants both from demand and supply perspectives, such as prices paid by consumers and reimbursement methods and rates for providers, are not generally available, and hence were not included in the analysis.

NOTES AND REFERENCES

1. See Robert A. Maxwell, *Health and Wealth: An International Study of Health Care Spending*, Lexington Books, Lexington, Massachusetts, 1981; Jan Blanpain, Bjorn Lindgren and Simone Sandier, *Comparaisons Internationales des Systèmes de Santé*, Centre de Recherche, d'Etude et de Documentation en Economie de la Santé, Paris, 1985; Joseph P. Newhouse, "Medical Care Expenditure: A Cross-National Survey", *Journal of Human Resources*, Winter 1977; and Robert E. Leu, "The Public-Private Mix and International Health Care Costs", in A.J. Culyer and Bengt Jönsson (eds.), *Public and Private Health Services*, Basil Blackwell Ltd., Oxford, 1986. A recent analysis of 18 countries for 1980 using health PPPs found elasticities of less than one. For a discussion of these results as well as the conceptual economic and econometric issues underlying such income elasticity estimations, see D. Parkin, A. McGuire and B. Yule, "Aggregate Health Care Expenditures and National Income: Is Health Care a Luxury Good?", *Journal of Health Economics*, Vol. 6, 1987.

2. However, the relationships are weaker in terms of changes than levels, both with regard to lower correlations and the fact that the significance levels of the overall relationships are weaker (e.g. for two of the three time periods, the relationship is significant at a 0.05 not 0.01 level of significance).

Chapter 8

TECHNOLOGY, DEMOGRAPHIC CHANGE
AND LONG-TERM CARE

Growth in expenditures over the past two decades has been due to increased utilisation and intensity of services and, to a lesser extent, to population growth. Changes in utilisation and intensity of services engendered by new medical technologies and different disease structures resulting from changing population composition could have important effects on future health care expenditures. Such changes will increasingly focus both demand and delivery systems on the provision of long-term care services for the chronically ill. Moreover, changes in population composition will also have important implications for financing these future expenditures. This chapter contains an analysis of these possible impacts. First, the difficulties of evaluating past as well as future impacts of technological change are discussed. Second, the financial implications of future demographic changes are analysed. Third, issues in the demand for, financing, and delivery of long-term care services are discussed.

Technology Change

Unfortunately, little is known at a cross-national level about the linkages between technological implementation, utilisation and intensity of services, health outcomes and costs. One study by Showstack *et al.*[1] analysed the cost and outcome implications of treating ten diagnoses (acute asthma, acute myocardial infarction, lung cancer, respiratory distress syndrome of the newborn, cataract excision, delivery (both cesarean section and vaginal), stapedectomy, total hip replacement, and kidney transplantation) in a 560-bed United States teaching facility. The authors collected detailed data for 1972, 1977 and 1982 and standardised these data for severity of illness among patients. The principal factor accounting for an increase in the average "quantity" of services per admission was the substitution of surgery for medical treatment for patients admitted for acute myocardial infarction, respiratory distress syndrome of the newborn, or delivery, and other intensive treatments of critically ill patients. Other changes in the styles of treatment contributed little to higher hospital costs. For example, in general the costs from the

substitution of new for older technologies were offset by shorter lengths of hospital stay. Costs, as a percentage of the average hospital bill, from the use of "little ticket" technologies such as laboratory tests were small (except for kidney transplants) and did not change much. They also found that charges for "big ticket" technologies, such as imaging services, increased only for certain diagnoses and generally (except for myocardial infarctions) were not a large percentage of the hospital bill. The study indicates that much of the debate on the cost implications of medical technology is too narrowly focused, since it frequently relates only to hardware costs and omits new surgical procedures and other services, the very factors found in this study to be responsible for increased treatment costs.

Of equal interest is that the study indicates that new clinical changes had little immediate effect on outcomes. On the other hand, another study found that the use of advanced medical technologies to keep high-risk, low birthweight infants alive resulted in a 16 per cent decrease in congenital abnormalities and developmental delays in infants to age one, although the question of whether these low birthweight children will eventually display higher rates of learning disabilities or mild neurological defects was unanswered[2]. Another study found that survival rates for patients in intensive care units vary less with medical technology use than with strong staff coordination[3]. These examples should be regarded as illustrative. While there are scattered pieces of evidence on the cost and outcome impacts of various medical technologies, the results are often partial, not systematically generalisable, and quite narrowly focused.

A recent study by the Institute of Medicine (IOM) of the United States National Academy of Sciences discusses many of the issues and problems in technology assessment[4]. Medical Technology is defined as "techniques, drugs, equipment, and procedures used by health care professionals in delivering medical care to individuals, and the systems with which such care is delivered". The study points out that current assessment activities are inconsistent in quality, poorly funded, that there are few assessments of cost-effectiveness or cost-benefit, and that assessments of ethical, legal, and other social implications are rare. The study indicates that the United States spent $384 billion on health care in 1984, $11.8 billion (3 per cent) on health research and development, but only $1.3 billion (0.3 per cent) on all health technology assessment.

The IOM study also discusses the factors that affect the adoption and abandonment of medical technologies. It indicates that there are ten factors that influence such diffusion. Four of these factors (prevailing theory, attributes of the innovation, features of the clinical situation, and presence of an advocate) are relatively insensitive to changes by policy-makers. Three others (environmental constraints and incentives, conduct and methods of evaluation, and channels of communication) are relatively susceptible to policy influences in the short run, and three others (practice setting, decision-making process, and characteristics of the potential adopter) may be sensitive to policy influences over time. The study further points out the importance of technology assessment for health care cost control as well as quality. The impacts of reimbursement systems both on technology implementation as well as reimbursement for technology assessment *per se* have important implications for quality and costs.

The IOM also reviewed medical technology assessment in other countries. It found that in all countries there is increasing concern for safety, efficacy, costs, and social and ethical issues. There are substantial cross-national variations in institutional arrangements to regulate and assess medical technology. Most countries have consistent national policies to evaluate the safety and efficacy of drugs; however, only the United States, Sweden, Japan and Canada have systematic regulations for devices. Sweden is one of the few countries with a national policy for the assessment of devices, equipment, and medical procedures. Coordination and collaboration is of critical importance. Unfortunately, information exchanges are hampered by the fact that most countries do not have coordinated and well-developed systems for medical technology assessment.

It is thus difficult to make generalisations about the future cost (or other) impacts of new technologies. Such technologies may be cost-inducing or cost-saving[5]. Much will depend on whether (and how) such technologies substitute for other older technologies as well as their impact on treatment setting, use of other services, and ultimately on health outcomes. These factors will in turn depend on research and development, planning, coverage, and reimbursement policies concerning evaluation and diffusion. Such policy development may also involve difficult ethical choices concerning rationing and stringent coverage conditions.

Demographic Change

Past growth in health expenditures was due to increased coverage of population groups under public and private programmes, demographic changes, general economic inflation, health care inflation in excess of general inflation, and increases in utilisation and intensity of services. Even assuming that universal coverage has been achieved, that efficiency-inducing reimbursement methods have been put into place, and that a plethora of other cost-inducing effects (e.g. increased supply of physicians) have been contained, countries are likely to face potentially large increases in health expenditures as a result of the combined effects of population ageing and technological change. The age structures of population, the costliness of certain new technologies, and the effects of these technologies and of environmental factors on ageing, could have significant effects on future health care costs and the ability of the productive population to support such future costs.

In analysing the future health expenditure and financing impacts of projected demographic changes, two important facts must be considered. First, health expenditures are highest for the very young and the very old. Second, from a financing perspective, what is of importance is not only the expenditures generated by vulnerable population groups, but also the size and hence the ability of the productive population to support such expenditures.

On the basis of recent demographic projections, most countries will face substantial ageing of their populations over the next 30 to 50 years, although this ageing will take place earlier and more rapidly in some countries, such as Japan, than in others. An OECD report on ageing populations[6] analyses these trends and their underlying demographic assumptions in detail. Table 42, based on that report, contains the percentages of the population 65 and over, total dependency ratios, and aged dependency ratios for 1980, 2010 and 2030 for the OECD countries. The percentage of the population aged 65 and over is projected to increase from an OECD average of 12.2 per cent in 1980 to 15.3 per cent in 2010 to 20.5 per cent in 2030. At higher age groups the proportional increases are even greater, so that between 1980 and 2030 the percentage of the population over 80 is expected to more than double, increasing from 2.1 per cent to 5 per cent. Given the expenditures associated with these elderly groups, these changes could have a substantial impact on health spending.

In order to analyse more precisely the effects of population ageing and growth on future health spending, information on the latter by age group is needed. Table 43 contains the ratio of spending for those aged 65 and over to those under 65 for the 16 OECD countries for which such data have been collected. Per capita health expenditures for the elderly are between 1.7 and 5.5 times the spending for the non-elderly, with a 16-country average of 4.0[7]. For the very old, expenditures are substantially higher.

An indication of the effects of future changes in population composition on future health expenditures, *ceteris paribus*, can be obtained for these 16 countries by calculating what total and per capita health expenditures would have been in 1980, if each country had faced

Table 42

TOTAL AND AGED DEPENDENCY RATIOS
1980, 2010, 2030

	Percentage of population 65 and over			Total dependency ratio			Aged dependency ratio		
	1980	2010	2030	1980	2010	2030	1980	2010	2030
Canada	9.51	14.61	22.39	48.13	46.62	66.48	14.09	21.42	37.28
France	13.96	16.26	21.76	56.84	50.83	64.43	21.89	24.53	35.78
Germany	15.51	20.35	25.82	50.79	50.47	68.69	23.39	30.62	43.56
Italy	13.45	17.28	21.92	54.89	48.62	61.06	20.83	25.68	35.30
Japan	9.10	18.62	19.97	48.40	58.63	59.48	13.50	29.53	31.85
United Kingdom	14.87	14.61	19.24	56.22	52.68	61.86	23.23	22.31	31.14
United States	11.29	12.79	19.49	51.08	47.19	62.35	17.06	18.83	31.65
Big Seven Average	12.53	16.36	21.51	52.34	50.72	63.48	19.14	24.70	35.22
Australia	9.62	12.59	18.22	53.54	48.18	59.15	14.77	24.70	35.22
Austria	15.47	17.45	22.82	56.23	52.50	66.63	24.17	26.62	38.03
Belgium	14.37	15.90	20.78	52.43	48.04	60.18	21.90	23.54	33.29
Denmark	14.41	16.67	22.56	54.46	45.71	61.51	22.25	24.29	36.44
Finland	11.98	16.76	23.78	47.67	48.35	67.13	17.69	24.86	39.74
Greece	13.14	16.77	19.49	56.13	53.27	57.95	20.52	25.70	30.79
Iceland	9.90	11.25	18.11	59.80	42.90	57.47	15.83	16.08	28.51
Ireland	10.72	11.08	14.74	69.97	47.33	54.09	18.22	16.33	22.71
Luxembourg	13.52	18.12	22.38	47.76	52.01	65.60	19.98	27.54	37.07
Netherlands	11.51	15.13	22.96	51.14	46.05	64.75	17.40	22.10	37.83
New Zealand	9.73	12.01	19.35	57.98	45.68	58.35	15.38	17.49	30.65
Norway	14.76	15.12	20.73	58.54	47.91	61.04	23.40	22.37	33.38
Portugal	10.17	14.13	18.24	58.56	51.13	57.34	16.12	21.36	28.70
Spain	10.85	15.53	19.64	58.08	47.79	58.42	17.16	22.95	31.11
Sweden	16.29	17.47	21.70	55.97	52.46	63.18	25.40	26.63	35.41
Switzerland	13.83	20.49	27.29	50.48	54.59	73.09	20.81	31.68	47.23
Turkey	4.74	5.52	8.92	78.12	49.02	54.33	8.45	8.22	13.77
OECD average	12.20	15.27	20.51	55.55	49.50	61.87	18.89	22.89	33.34

Source: The Social Policy Implications of Ageing Populations, OECD, Paris, forthcoming.

its projected population compositions of 2010 and 2030, respectively. This is equivalent to projecting what health expenditures would be in 2010 and 2030 in 1980-base-year dollars, holding constant medical practice patterns, delivery arrangements, reimbursement effects, health outcomes, expenditures on the elderly versus the non-elderly, etc.[8].

Table 43 also displays for each of the 16 countries the percentage changes in total and per capita health spending implied by age structure changes in 2010 and 2030. The 2010 population structure results in a 16-country average overall spending increase of 17 per cent and a per capita increase of 7 per cent. This would suggest that, holding all other factors constant, total spending would increase at a compound annual rate of 0.52 per cent, while per capita spending would increase at a compound annual rate of 0.22 per cent. Given the decline in the total dependency ratio and the relatively small increase in the aged dependency ratio, under reasonable assumptions of economic growth, financing these services would not appear on average to pose a serious problem.

As would be expected, the figures for individual countries show significant variation. Belgium, Denmark, France, Ireland, Italy, Sweden, the United Kingdom and the United States would not appear to face major new per capita expenditure increases due to population growth and ageing, since per capita spending would increase by 5 per cent or less. On the other hand, Japan, Canada, Finland and Switzerland would appear to be facing new financing burdens, as per capita health expenditures increase by 10 per cent or more with most of the increase due to increases in the numbers and proportion of the elderly population. Japan and Switzerland would appear to be facing significant increases in their financing burdens, since their aged dependency and total dependency ratios increase significantly. The increased financing burden should be less in Finland and Canada, where increases in aged dependency ratios are somewhat offset by declines in total dependency ratios.

The story is rather different for 2030. Between 1980 and 2030 average health expenditures for the 16 countries will increase by 31 per cent (compound annual growth rate of 0.54), while per capita spending will increase by 19 per cent (compound annual growth rate of 0.35). Much of this increase occurs in the 20 years between 2010 and 2030, as total and per capita expenditures increase by 10 and 12 per cent, respectively, as many countries feel the full effects of population ageing. These expenditure increases would even be

Table 43

HEALTH EXPENDITURES BY AGE AND GROWTH IN SPENDING
BY 2010 AND 2030

Country	Ratio of per capita health spending on those age 65 and over to those under 65	Percentage increase in spending (b)					
		1980 - 2010		2010 - 2030		1980 - 2030	
		Total	Per Capita	Total	Per Capita	Total	Per Capita
Australia	4.9	50	9	33	15	99	24
Belgium	1.7	-1	1	-1	3	-1	4
Canada	4.5	46	13	31	18	90	34
Denmark	4.1	-4	5	0	20	-4	17
Finland	5.5	18	14	11	18	30	35
France	2.4	11	3	5	6	16	9
Germany	2.6	-3	6	-8	7	-10	13
Ireland	4.5	22	1	16	9	41	10
Italy	2.2	1	4	-4	5	-3	9
Japan	4.8	40	27	-2	3	36	31
Netherlands	4.5	17	9	13	18	32	29
New Zealand	4.2	31	6	24	17	62	24
Sweden	5.5 (a)	2	3	9	11	11	14
Switzerland	3.6 (a)	16	13	4	12	20	26
United Kingdom	4.3	2	0	12	10	15	10
United States	3.9 (a)	27	3	23	14	56	18
Average	4.0	17	7	10	12	31	19
Compound annual rate of growth		0.52	0.22	0.48	0.57	0.54	0.35

Notes: a) Ratio of total health spending of those aged 65 and over to those below age 65. For other countries the ratio reflects public spending only.

b) Calculations are based on the assumption that the ratios of per capita total health spending of those aged 65 and over to those below 65 in 1980 are the same as the ratios presented here.

Sources: The Social Policy Implications of Ageing Populations, OECD, Paris, forthcoming.
Data for the United States are OECD estimates based on preliminary 1984 data supplied by the U.S. Health Care Financing Administration.
Data for Italy are from G. Lojacono, Study on the Evaluation of Cost/Effectiveness of Alternative Strategies for the Health Care of the Elderly, World Health Organisation, 1985, Part C, p. 35.
Data for Switzerland are from P. Gygi and A. Frei: Le Domaine de la Santé Publique en Suisse, en 1980, Basle, 1982.
Data for New Zealand are from Frances Sutton, Age Distribution of Vote Health Expenditure 1979/80, Department of Health, Wellington, 1983.
Data for Finland provided by the Planning Secretariat of the Ministry of Social Affairs and Health, Helsinki.

higher if differential expenditure weights were available for the very young and the very old.

From an individual country perspective, over the entire 50-year time period Australia, Canada, Denmark, Finland, Japan, the Netherlands, New Zealand, Switzerland and the United States could be facing significant new financing burdens on the basis of population ageing alone, as per capita health expenditures could increase in excess of 15 per cent, or at compound rates of over 0.3 percentage point per year. The financial implications would appear to be the largest for Canada, Finland and Japan, which could face increases in per capita expenditures in excess of 30 per cent or at compound rates of over 0.5 percentage point per year. On the other hand, Belgium, France, Ireland, Italy and the United Kingdom would appear to be facing the smallest increases in per capita spending, as expenditures increase by 10 per cent or less, or at compound annual rates of less than 0.2 percentage point.

The financing burden of health expenditures falls mainly on the working population. As such, the ability of countries to finance these increased expenditures resulting from population ageing (as well as those emanating from general population growth) will depend on changes in the relative size of the productive population as reflected in dependency ratios, as well as labour force participation rates, unemployment rates and productivity. As would be expected, those countries facing potentially large increases in per capita expenditures also face large increases in their aged dependency ratios and, to a lesser extent, in their total dependency ratios. While the average aged dependency ratio for the OECD countries increases by less than 80 per cent over the 50-year period, the aged dependency ratios of Australia, Canada, Finland, Japan, and Switzerland will increase by some 150 per cent. The increases in aged dependency ratios in the low expenditure increase countries are on the order of 50 per cent. All OECD countries except Iceland, Ireland, Portugal and Turkey face increases in their total dependency ratios, with Finland, Canada, Luxembourg and Switzerland facing the largest increases.

Also of importance from a financing perspective is the timing of the increases in spending over the 50-year period. Of those countries facing the largest increases in per capita expenditures, the compound annual increases in per capita spending for Denmark, the Netherlands, New Zealand and the United States are generally at least twice as large in the 2010-2030 period than from 1980-2010. On the other hand, the increases in spending faced by Japan mostly occur in the 1980-2010 period, and for Canada, Finland and Switzerland are relatively evenly divided over both periods.

In summary, and setting aside significant differences among countries, it appears likely, *ceteris paribus*, that by the year 2030 OECD countries will be faced on average with total health expenditures some 30 per cent higher, and per capita health expenditures some 20 per cent higher as a result of population ageing. At current levels of expenditure, this represents an additional burden of 2 to 3 per cent of GDP. However, this presumes that all other potentially cost-inducing factors are held constant. Of course there are many imponderables to this kind of analysis, and it is difficult to judge at this stage how much strain on resources will result from the additional requirements of health programmes. Given adequate growth in productivity and employment, the aggregate economic burden need not prove insuperable. But it could require significant re-allocations of resources from other competing goals and a political willingness to provide the mechanisms which will accommodate such a shift in priorities.

Long-Term Care

Ageing populations, life-sustaining technological changes, changing morbidity and disability patterns, and changing demographic and economic conditions (family size, mobility, decline of the extended family, working women) are likely to result in increased demands for formal long-term care services. Unfortunately, while long-term care is quite topical, at a comparative international level there appears to be more rhetoric than fact, a dearth of universally accepted definitions, little available data on needs assessment or features of delivery systems, and little behavioural response analysis.

In order to discuss long-term care, one must define it. The most common approach employed in the past to distinguish long-term from acute care was to employ a time duration cut-off (e.g. long-term care stays in a hospital are those that exceed 30 days). From an epidemiological perspective activity limitations are a measure of long-term care needs. Others have focused on functional disability, as it more closely approximates behaviour. Indeed the debate here is much the same as in the previous discussion on health outcomes. No one measure can satisfactorily capture and isolate the numerous factors affecting long-term needs, and no one measure is sufficient for analysing the implications of alternative policy changes.

Two definitions reported by Weissert[9] are useful in defining both the long-term care population and the services needed:

- "The long-term care population consists of all persons, regardless or age or diagnosis, who, because of a chronic condition, require or receive human help in personal care, mobility, household activities, or home-administered health care services. Personal care includes eating, continence, transferring (e.g. moving from bed to chair, or bed to floor), toileting, dressing, and bathing. Mobility includes walking and going outside. Household activities include meal preparation, money management, shopping and chores, excluding yard work. Home-administered health care services include injections, dressings, physical therapy, and other health care services".

- "Long-term care consists of those services designed to provide diagnosis, preventative, therapeutic, rehabilitative, supportive, and maintenance services for individuals of all age groups who have chronic physical and/or mental impairments, in a variety of institutional and noninstitutional health care settings, including the home, with the goals of promoting optimum levels of physical, social and psychological functioning".

These definitions point up the various behavioural and service aspects of long-term care: functional disability, chronic illness, human assistance, and social, psychological and medical institutional and non-institutional services. Clearly, from a public programme perspective long-term care goes well beyond health programmes and includes housing, social and family assistance, pensions, and social welfare services. While the principal populations needing these services are aged, non-aged individuals also need long-term care services. Nevertheless, even if future risks of disability and chronic morbidity remain unchanged (a questionable assumption), large increases in the demand for long-term care services will occur as a result of the higher incidence of chronic disease in the larger cohorts moving into older ages and increases in the duration of illness associated with increases in life expectancy[10].

There are wide disparities in the financing, coverage and delivery of long-term care services across OECD countries. Studies by the International Social Security Association and the United States Senate document substantial differences in these features[11]. Both studies found large differences in institutionalisation rates and the use of home health services. Use rates for medically-oriented residential facilities tended to be higher in Canada and the United States, while use rates for non-medically-oriented residential facilities were much higher in Europe. The Senate study also found wide variations in the use of publicly funded home care services, with the highest use rates in the United Kingdom and Sweden and the lowest in Switzerland, Canada and Germany.

Benefits under formal health and social service systems differ significantly across countries. Frequently, the social service aspects of long-term care are not covered as part of the formal health care financing and delivery system, and serious problems of coordination between medical and social service delivery systems exist. However, in other countries there are few coordination problems. In addition to coverage of non-medical institutional (including strictly residential) services, a number of countries cover home help aids, and in several countries family members can be reimbursed for providing such services. However, much care is also currently provided through informal non-market family arrangements. Many countries also provide cash grants to disabled elderly individuals.

Financing and delivery systems also differ significantly. In the Scandinavian countries, the United Kingdom and the Netherlands, long-term care is almost exclusively provided by the public sector, directly or indirectly, while in the United States, Germany and Switzerland there is substantially more private sector involvement in both financing and provision.

Needs assessment is by no means simple, and in a number of countries there is substantial unmet need. The Scandinavian countries, the Netherlands, the United Kingdom and some Canadian provinces have formal screening mechanisms, and Denmark uses multidisciplinary assessment committees. Nevertheless, the limited available data suggest that in most countries there is still substantial inappropriate use of hospital and other medically-oriented institutional services by the elderly. Some of this is due to shortages of nursing home beds and/or community support services. The Swiss have recently removed coverage of hospital stays for social reasons. On the other hand, there are still large numbers of individuals in the community with disabilities serious enough to require institutionalisation. For example, in the United States for each person in a nursing home, there are two individuals living in the community with comparable levels of disability.

It is clear from the above discussion that the design of policies for the financing and delivery of long-term care services are fraught with conceptual as well as ethical difficulties. Furthermore, such policies must be coordinated with those in the acute care area. In the following chapter, these policy choices are discussed.

NOTES AND REFERENCES

1. Jonathan A. Showstack *et al.*, "The Role of Changing Clinical Practices In the Rising Cost of Hospital Care", *The New England Journal of Medicine*, Vol. 313, No. 19, Nov. 7, 1985.

2. *Special Report: The Perinatal Program - What Has Been Learned*, Robert Wood Johnson Foundation, Princeton, New Jersey, 1985.

3. William Knaus *et al.*, "An Evaluation of Outcome From Intensive Care In Major Medical Centers", *Annals of Internal Medicine*, Vol. 104, No. 3, March 1986.

4. *Assessing Medical Technologies*, Institute of Medicine, National Academy Press, Washington, D.C., 1985.

5. See Jack Meyer, "The Implications of Ageing Populations for Health Care Policy and Expenditures", internal working paper, OECD, Paris, 1984; and *The Social Policy Implications of Ageing Populations*, OECD, Paris, forthcoming.

6. *The Social Policy Implications of Ageing Populations*, *Ibid.*

7. These ratios should be interpreted with caution since they are not completely comparable in terms of the items included.

8. These are not very realistic assumptions; however, the methodology provides a measure of the potential expenditure effects of population ageing alone.

9. William G. Weissert, "Estimating the Long-Term Care Population: Prevalence Rates and Selected Characteristics", *Health Care Financing Review*, Summer 1985, p. 84.

10. See Bryan Luce, Korbin Liu and Kenneth G. Manton, "Estimating the Long-Term Care Population and Its Use of Services", *Long-Term Care and Social Security*, International Social Security Association, Geneva, 1984.

11. *Long-Term Care for the Elderly Provided Within the Framework of Health Care Schemes*, International Social Security Association, XXIInd General Assembly, Montreal, 2-12 September 1986; and *Long-Term Care in Western Europe and Canada: Implications for the United States*, Special Committee on Ageing, United States Senate, Washington, D.C., 1984.

Chapter 9

CONCLUSIONS FOR POLICY

The earlier chapters of this report concentrated on comparisons of health outcomes, health service utilisation, and health expenditures in OECD countries. This final chapter is concerned with health care policy. The first section of the chapter sets out the principal difficulties in health policy formulation. It is followed by a short discussion of the goals of public policy and a taxonomy of various policy measures which can be used to achieve them. A brief final section brings together the main policy conclusions.

Difficulties in Health Policy Formulation

It is useful, before discussing the goals of health care policy reforms and the range of policy options, to summarise the basic difficulties underlying health policy formulation. These include:

- Health care outcomes and hence efficiency and effectiveness are not measurable;
- Access and/or equality of access is difficult to define and measure (e.g. financial access, physical access, equality of access versus equality of outcomes, etc.);
- Knowledge about appropriateness of medical care is extremely limited;
- There are few behavioural studies of reimbursement, delivery systems organisation, and supply response that are readily generalisable;
- Health care systems cannot be treated in isolation of social service systems, lifestyles, and environmental factors;
- Quality is difficult to define, rarely monitored, and one of the most neglected areas of international comparisons.

Thus, governments are unable, by any means fully, to evaluate the effects of the many billions of dollars spent on health care[1]. In part this situation is able to continue politically because of the publics' general satisfaction in most countries with their health systems[2].

The information presented in this report, as well as numerous other studies, raises a number of large and important questions at the national level and also across countries:

- How is value for money to be measured in the case of health care?
- Are observed significant differences in health expenditures reflected in differences in health outcomes, quality, amenities, or efficiency?
- Which aspects of health systems provide the most value for money, and which the least?
- To what extent does the observed rapid growth of health expenditures reflect the growth of incomes and demand, the development of new technologies, the way in which health care is financed, or the pressure of supplying professionals?
- Why does the availability and use of hospital and physician services differ so much, and what are the expenditure and outcome implications?
- To what extent can increased health expenditure, as compared with other measures outside the health care system, improve life expectancy, enhance the quality of life, and reduce death rates?
- What are the essential characteristics of the 4 or 5 per cent of people who account for half of all health expenditures, and can these expenditures be controlled?

Unfortunately precise answers cannot be given to these questions. To some extent this is a difficulty associated with all questions of social policy choice. Decision-makers never have all the information they would like to have. However, several basic institutional factors in the health sector make health care policy choices intrinsically more difficult than those for other sectors. Among these are: the interposition of a major industry motivated by both pecuniary and non-pecuniary incentives between the consumer and the financing entity; the inability of consumers or financing entities to evaluate the benefits versus cost of services purchased; public and private third-party insurers which insulate consumers and producers from the economic consequences of their decisions; and the importance of lifestyles, consumption of non-medical public and private services, and general environmental factors in determining both the need and the use of health services.

Nevertheless, fiscal pressures combined with the considerable political sensitivity on the part of unions, consumers, providers and insurers require policy-makers to make choices in a world of second best alternatives.

Issues for Policy

The main objectives of health care policy in all OECD countries are redistribution, social protection, and assuring the efficient production and consumption of health services. Such policies are undertaken as a result of market failure in the health sector as well as normative societal judgements concerning "equal access" to necessary care, irrespective of ability to pay and differences in "need".

Current problems and policy recommendations concerning access as well as the financing and delivery of health care are related to perceived failure to meet these objectives fully. Given the difficulties of measuring access and efficiency, much of the present policy debate is driven by value judgements, conventional wisdom, and short-run budgetary considerations. For example, with regard to efficiency it has been shown that one of the principal factors responsible for the growth in real health care expenditures has been increased utilisation and intensity of services. Yet, it is less clear exactly what increases in utilisation and intensity of service mean, and how specific features of health systems have contributed to such growth.

Measuring access is even more difficult, because in addition to serious measurement problems, significant normative judgements are involved. Distinctions can be made between physical and financial access, and equality of access versus equality of outcomes. In most OECD countries over 95 per cent of the population has financial access to hospital care. In most countries usage by the poor has increased substantially following the introduction of public programmes. Nevertheless, despite access, differences in relative use rates between the poor and non-poor have not changed much in some countries; there are still substantial differences in mortality rates and life expectancy; and there are concerns about the underutilisation by certain socio-economic groups[3]. Needs and/or unmet needs of various population subgroups are difficult to define and measure, and few data are available for comparative studies.

A further complication is that individual (or groups of) policies may promote conflicting objectives. Policies to assure efficiency in the delivery or consumption of services may have adverse effects on equity, and conversely. In the extreme this can result in two-tier medicine, and raises difficult equity and ethical questions about whether the rich should be able to purchase new life-saving technologies which are not covered by the public programmes. In some countries discussions have focused on adequate access to high quality but not necessarily the top quality. Is there a concept of "quality second class care", and if so, how should it be defined? In other countries access to the same exhaustive set of benefits for the entire population is seen as a fundamental aspect of the welfare state. Despite these apparent differences, however, all countries place some limits on service coverage, and upper income (and other) individuals are not precluded from expressing their demand for non-covered services through private market mechanisms. Yet, the question of placing limits on overall societal consumption of health services has been raised along with the difficult question of the justification for singling out health care as the sole (legal) service for which individuals are not allowed to express their preferences through free market mechanisms. These conflicts and questions cannot be resolved analytically. Clearly societal choices expressed through the political systems of the various countries will have to resolve this issue.

The consideration of health care policies can focus both on revenues and expenditures. Ideally, policies should be discussed in terms of financial effects, access effects, quality impacts, and their effects on health outcomes. It can be useful also to consider the trade-offs between expenditures on health in comparison with other public programmes and private consumption or private investment. These trade-offs have been discussed in other publications[4] and hence are not discussed here. Furthermore, because much of the current debate on health policy emphasizes efficiency and cost containment, while physical and financial access have generally been achieved in most countries, the discussion of policy options below focuses on achieving efficiency rather than on major new expansions of health services. Nevertheless, the impacts of policies on access of consumers, delivery systems, quality and outcomes are also discussed.

Policies can be focused on the demand side, the supply side, and on financing. They can affect all of the participants in the health care system: consumers, medical care providers, private and public insurers, governmental entities, employers, trade unions, and charitable institutions. A general taxonomy of policy objectives under economic constraints would include the following: restrain (or promote efficient) health care prices, reduce (or promote efficient) utilisation of services, narrow programme boundaries, and improve financing.

Policies designed to restrain health care prices focus on setting prospective payment rates, establishing relative price levels (within and across provider type) that promote the efficient use of resources, indexation of increases to general (as opposed to health sector-specific) inflation or input prices, aggregating ("bundling") services to remove incentives for providers to fragment their billings, and the use of market power through competitive bidding to promote competition. In addition to the relative and absolute prices and their inherent efficiency incentives, the impacts of price reforms on the quantity and hence total expenditure sides are critical. Thus, establishing "efficient" prices by setting rates prospectively is not sufficient for controlling total costs, because there may be serious implications for the quantity side depending on the unit of payment (per day, per stay, per case), and monitoring of quantities is thus very important. Similarly, the interaction across provider types cannot be ignored, because price control policies on one set of providers (e.g. ambulatory care physicians) may result in more costly substitutions of other services (e.g. increased hospitalisation). Policies to restrain utilisation may well be needed as a concomitant to price control policies.

The impact of price restraint on access, quality, and health outcomes is also important. If prices are set at levels below the real resource costs borne by the medical care provider in efficiently producing the service, and assuming that the resulting deficits are not eliminated through public subsidies or cost-shifting, then in the long run providers will react by refusing to participate, reducing quality, or reducing the intensity of services. However, if there are substantial inefficiencies in service production, and competitive (or other regulatory) pressures prevail, price restraint can improve efficiency without harming quality, access or outcomes.

Over the past several years many countries have restrained prices for health services, affecting particularly hospitals, physicians, and pharmaceuticals[5]. Many of the measures taken have been based solely on budgetary grounds and have not been targeted to overall reform of reimbursement systems. Such measures include freezes or indexation of hospital reimbursements, physician fee schedules, and pharmaceutical reimbursements. In the process there has been relatively little evaluation of the impacts of such policies on quality, access, outcomes or increased service provision that can offset potential savings from price controls. However, in a number of countries either major reforms or basic elements of reform have been the principal elements of price restraint policies. The DRG-based prospective payment system in the United States and the prospectively-set global budgets in France are examples of price restraint policies embodying incentive reforms. While it is too soon to evaluate the French reforms, the preliminary evidence from the United States indicates substantial reductions in length of stay, hospital utilisation, and expenditures. Assessing the impact on quality has been difficult, however[6]. Limitations on hospital reimbursements in Belgium have been accompanied by strong incentives to convert excess hospital beds into nursing home beds. On the other hand, most physician price restraints embody simply the freezing of fees, with no basic incentive reforms. However, several countries such as the United States, the Netherlands, Japan and France have been attempting to adjust relative fee levels to promote appropriate allocational incentives in the provision of physician services. Unfortunately, there is little empirical evidence on the effects of such changes on the use of specific physician

and other health services or on the effects on overall spending and health outcomes.

Some countries have focused their reimbursement activities on high volume services. For example, data from the United States indicate that the insertion of prosthetic lenses, the extraction of lenses, the insertion of pacemakers, prostatectomy and arthroplasty and the replacement of hips account for substantial amounts of total expenditure on the elderly, as well as over 70 per cent of the total inpatient demand for such services[7]. Other countries have focused their efforts on high volume pharmaceuticals and the use of lower cost generic equivalents. Competitive bidding and bulk purchasing, as in the United Kingdom for laundry and food services for hospitals or in the United States under several State Medicaid programmes for hospital services, eyeglasses and hearing aids are also examples of the use of reimbursement mechanisms to induce efficiency and reduce costs.

Policies to reduce utilisation can focus on consumers through cost-sharing, providers through alternative delivery arrangements and health planning and delivery system controls, and consumers and providers through administrative reviews. Cost-sharing is currently employed as a financing and/or resource allocation mechanism in most OECD countries. Philosophical issues aside, the key questions regarding its further use as a cost-containment mechanism are whether changes in cost-sharing reduce consumption of services over the long run, and their effect on health status and hence long-run costs. A question arises as to the potential effectiveness of cost-sharing as an allocational mechanism, and its potential conflict with distributional objectives, since some 5 per cent of individuals account for half of all spending.

There is a major debate at present about the effects of cost-sharing in terms of its effect on expenditures as well as on health status[8]. There appears to be a strong feeling in several European countries that the introduction of cost-sharing results in an initial drop in utilisation, then followed by increases back to the original consumption trends. Much of the behavioural information on cost-sharing comes from the Rand Health Insurance Experiment in the United States. Effects on expenditures and on health outcomes have been analysed. With respect to expenditures, those individuals facing cost-sharing used fewer outpatient and hospital services. In both cases, the cost per treatment between those with and those without cost-sharing was similar, the basic reductions occurring in the number of episodes of care[9]. Similarly, Rand found that cost-sharing relative to free care substantially reduced the use of hospital emergency department services for less serious diagnoses[10]. With respect to health status, of ten health measures initially analysed for adults, free care was associated with improvements only for corrected vision and high blood pressure, and did not affect the health status of the average enrollee. In other words, cost-sharing relative to free care did appear to affect individuals with certain conditions that are easy to diagnose and have well-established treatment patterns (e.g. myopia, hypertension), but in most cases did not negatively affect outcomes[11].

In practice virtually all OECD countries require some cost-sharing, at least for prescription drugs. As mentioned above, in some countries cost-sharing is regarded as inconsistent with fundamental philosophical approaches to social welfare. Nevertheless, in most European countries cost-sharing is quite nominal (e.g. DM 5 per hospital day for up to 14 days in Germany, BF 168 per hospital day for the non-poor in Belgium, Y 300 per day for up to 60 days in Japan) and there are relatively low catastrophic limits or significant exclusions exist.

In general it does not appear that, except for pharmaceuticals, cost-sharing has been used in a major way as a resource allocation device in many OECD countries. Even in countries such as France and Japan where copayment and/or coinsurance rates appear substantial (e.g. 20-25 per cent), low limits on total out-of-pocket costs and exclusions for many categories of cases or individuals result in relatively small out-of-pocket costs and, probably, limited behavioural impacts. While such limitations may be philosophically consistent with the basic precepts of the welfare state, it could be argued that given the relatively small negative effects on health outcomes, such policies are inconsistent with allocational efficiency, and that income redistribution to needy groups could be more efficiently carried out through cash grants than through limitations on cost-sharing[12].

Alternative delivery arrangements, such as Health Maintenance Organisations (HMOs) and Preferred Provider Organisations (PPOs), can reduce utilisation by making medical care providers financially responsible for their decisions and by limiting consumer choice of provider to those willing to abide by the rules of the organisation. Such arrangements rely on market incentives rather than insurers' controls or government regulations.

A plethora of new delivery arrangements has the potential to reduce expenditures through the more efficient provision of services. Among these new arrangements are: diagnostic imaging centres, pain clinics, freestanding cancer centres, birth centres, hospices, home health care, wellness programmes, rehabilitation centres, ambulatory care centres, physician group practices, HMOs, PPOs, freestanding ambulatory and surgery centres, alcohol and drug abuse centres, mental health facilities, nursing homes, and independent clinical laboratories. Expenditures can be reduced through incentives for efficient provision (HMOs), reduced reimbursements for volume guarantees (PPOs), through the substitution of less medically intensive levels of institutional care (nursing homes for hospitals), outpatient for inpatient care (freestanding clinics of various types, home health care) or through the prevention of illness (e.g. wellness programmes).

The savings potential of many of these new delivery arrangements will depend on whether they are substitutes or add-ons to existing services, and concomitantly on methods of reimbursement and coverage rules. HMOs and ambulatory surgery centres have been shown to lead to significant reductions in hospital expenditures. There has been considerable interest in HMOs because for a fixed expenditure per year per enrollee, the HMO is responsible for all care. Hence, HMOs have incentives not only to limit spending but to keep enrollees healthy. HMOs have grown rapidly in the United States, with enrolment increasing from 5.7 million in 1975 to 19 million in 1985, and it has been suggested that enrolments may increase to 50 million by 1990. Research on HMOs has shown that the main reason that HMOs are 10-40 per cent cheaper than fee-for-service medicine is that hospitalisation, largely because of fewer admissions, is reduced. The evidence is less clear concerning the competitive effects of HMOs in eliciting cost-containing responses from conventional insurers and fee-for-service providers. Questions have also been raised in terms of whether HMOs enroll healthier individuals and the technical capacity of governments to establish capitation rates for high-risk groups. Furthermore, some studies indicate that although HMOs cause a once and for all reduction in costs, their rates of cost increase are not substantially different from those in the fee-for-service sector, suggesting that HMOs implement new technologies as rapidly as do non-HMOs[13]. Moreover, there have been few studies that compare HMO performance in terms of outcomes. One important question about the future relative performance of HMOs concerns the degree of efficiency incentives in the non-HMO sector. Luft[14] points out that much of the information on HMO performance and behaviour is based on a time period when there were few, if any, pressures for cost containment and efficiency. He further indicates that there is growing evidence of conventional insurers performing as well as HMOs and raises the question of whether the past relative performance of HMOs will be observed in the current more competitive medical care environment. Nevertheless, from *a priori* economic and health incentive perspectives, HMOs would appear to provide appropriate incentives for efficiency, whether in a highly regulated or a market-oriented health care system.

Direct regulation of the delivery system through planning activities that ration new technologies, limit capital expenditures on facilities and equipment, and regulate the overall supply of medical care personnel can also affect the utilisation of services. Such policies can also have significant effects on access, costs and quality of services. Similarly, administrative review procedures such as prior authorisation for hospital admissions, second surgical opinions, concurrent reviews, post-treatment reviews, and retrospective claims reviews can all affect utilisation, quality and place of delivery of services. Such reviews can be required by paying entities, governmental or private, or be an inherent feature of alternative delivery systems.

Countries are dealing with a variety of delivery system

reforms to reduce expenditures. Virtually all OECD countries are restricting medical school enrolments, and in some countries new physicians are able to receive insurance billing numbers only for underserved areas. Countries are trying to reduce excess hospital beds in a variety of ways, including conversion to long-term care beds and in some cases (e.g. Belgium, Germany, Switzerland, the Netherlands) by limiting costly intensive-care beds. Several countries (e.g. Japan) are developing more effective planning systems and technology assessment is receiving increased attention. Countries are putting more effort into prevention, lifestyles, and measuring outcomes. Increased attention is also being devoted to utilisation review, both from cost and quality perspectives. Tougher reimbursement systems require monitoring of utilisation both for appropriateness and to prevent fraud and abuse. The United States Congress tied enactment of the DRG system to the implementation of a new utilisation review system (e.g. Professional Review Organisations). Nevertheless, in many OECD countries formal quality assurance systems are weak or non-existent. Truly effective cost-containment can be achieved only if quality of care and health outcomes do not suffer.

Narrowing programme boundaries through changes in eligibility standards or benefits covered can also reduce expenditures. Affluent groups can be dropped from coverage and marginal benefits eliminated or reduced. In certain countries, more affluent groups are given the option to buy public or private coverage with little or no public subsidy. Other countries have reduced benefits in areas perceived as marginal (spa treatments, certain pharmaceuticals) and/or have provided incentives for the use of cost-effective preventive services and healthy lifestyles. These activities are taking place through social insurance systems, public health programmes, and direct regulation of individual behaviour (e.g. seat belt laws, smoking restrictions in public buildings, etc.). Beneficiary freedom of choice of medical care providers can also be reduced to encourage use of lower cost providers. Critical issues here are whether only public or overall health care costs are reduced, and the extent to which benefit, eligibility, and freedom of choice changes reduce necessary access and/or result in increased future costs or lost productivity.

There have however been few, if any, major changes in hospital or physician service benefits. Marginal new benefits such as hospice care have been added in some countries and new therapies such as liver and heart transplants have been covered for certain population groups. While there do not appear to be substantial changes in benefits covered, countries are increasingly adding economic efficiency criteria to the "medically necessary" criteria that are generally employed to establish coverage of new procedures. Increased attention is also being devoted to denying coverage for medical procedures that are no longer deemed to be medically effective.

Limiting freedom of choice of physicians or hospitals is prevalent. Several countries (e.g. the United Kingdom, Denmark, Spain, Ireland) currently limit choice of either generalist or specialist physicians. In the California State Medicaid programme only those hospitals accepted on the basis of a competitive bidding process may be used by programme beneficiaries. Limitations of freedom of choice in terms of using physicians as gatekeepers, guaranteeing medical care providers volume in exchange for discounts, and/or limiting coverage to only lower cost providers are all features that are inherent in efficient alternative delivery systems such as HMOs. However, policy changes in this area must carefully weigh the potential for cost-saving against access, quality and outcome concerns as well as consumer preferences.

Health care expenditures can be reduced or revenues enhanced through a variety of financing changes. Overall budget controls can be put into place by establishing a closed-ended annual appropriation. Such appropriations can be established to limit total health spending, national government spending or spending for particular types of services. The issues here are the allocation of the total in a way that promotes efficient resource use and the potential for cost-shifting. If costs are shifted to local governments or consumers, total medical costs or indeed total governmental costs may not be controlled. Similarly, expenditures can be closed-ended through health care voucher approaches, such as that proposed in the United States whereby individuals would be given a voucher of fixed value to purchase private health insurance. By purchasing from the most efficient entity or delivery system, the consumer gets more services and the government's financial liability is limited to the voucher amount. The key issues with vouchers, like HMOs, are establishing the capitation amounts, the series of problems of adverse selection if the government remains the insurer of last resort, the necessary regulation of the private sector, and the potential for cost-shifts to beneficiaries and local governments.

Other financing approaches that increase revenues include raising existing or introducing new taxes, raising or introducing premiums, and eliminating tax subsidies for the purchase of insurance and/or medical care services. The issues here are twofold. One is the allocational, distributional and overall macro-economic impact of such changes. The second is that revenue enhancement does little to control overall health care costs or impose efficiency on delivery systems. Thus, to the extent that rising health care costs are deemed to be a problem on allocational efficiency grounds, revenue enhancements do little to deal with the problem.

The policy measures discussed above have focused on acute care. While many of the same generic types of options have been discussed for long-term care, certain medical, social and financial aspects of chronically ill patients necessitate a separate policy discussion. In particular, the needs of patients are often social rather than purely medical. Long-term care may entail simply maintaining a patient in his or her current state, slowing the rate of deterioration, or merely providing aid and comfort as the patient's condition steadily and inevitably deteriorates. Financing is also more complex because it is difficult to budget for and predict long-term care needs; and currently there is a great deal of non-market production provided by family members.

Much of the current policy debate about long-term care focuses on needs assessment, efficiency, delivery systems and financing. A study by ISSA found that the two most pressing policy concerns of the countries surveyed were the rising costs and excessive use of institutional long-term care services[15]. As a result, much of the current debate concerns defining patients' needs and matching those needs with the most efficient mode of service delivery. In some countries there has been a considerable effort to develop channelling agencies and case coordinators to manage patients' overall service needs. There is much emphasis on de-institutionalisation and home care. Yet it is clear that for some patients with given disability levels and medical needs, institutional care is more appropriate. Much of the effort involves designing appropriate packages of medical, social and other support services to maintain self-sufficiency. New types of services such as hospices can in many cases be more humane and less costly ways of treating the terminally ill. Some discussion has focused on reimbursement, especially prospective reimbursement and capitation approaches. Yet such methods applied to chronic as compared with acute care patients raise special conceptual and operational problems. Since the health status of patients with chronic disabilities does not necessarily improve (indeed it may continue to deteriorate) and many of the quality assurance mechanisms inherent in the delivery of acute care are lacking (e.g. extensive physician involvement), strong reimbursement restrictions and total expenditure limits may reduce quality.

There has been much discussion and some activity concerning the development of appropriate delivery systems. As mentioned above, a number of countries are actively attempting to convert acute care hospital beds into nursing home beds. Hospices, outpatient clinics for rehabilitation and chronic pain management, and outpatient mental health care are developing both through public and private sector efforts. Various voluntary service and other innovative arrangements for delivering care (e.g. having the mailman checking on elderly individuals living alone) are being scrutinised.

There is also much policy debate on the financing of long-term care. Given the potentially large increase in demand due to both population ageing and changes in social structures, there are major concerns about paying for such services in the future. In the United States there is considerable interest in private sector financing of long-term care. Private long-term care insurance, individual medical retirement accounts, and reverse equity mortgages are all being studied as potential private sector solutions to the financing of long-term care.

There is also much discussion concerning discontinuing medical treatment for terminally-ill patients. Such discussions raise difficult moral and ethical issues. The rights of terminally-ill patients to request discontinuation of further medical treatment have been fairly widely recognised. However, there is currently an emotional debate over the withholding of fluids and nutrients from such patients. For the most part decisions to discontinue care have been left to individuals and their physicians, although in the cases of specific technologies such as renal dialysis and organ transplants, government decisions have either implicitly (e.g. through limiting the total available number of dialysis machines) or explicitly (e.g. through excluding chronic alcoholics from liver transplants) excluded certain individuals from coverage. However, ageing populations with increased disabilities combined with technological changes that even at present allow machines to substitute for various organs, could put increased pressure on governments to make explicit decisions about rationing care through their medical coverage criteria.

Some countries are focusing on prevention and fostering medical research to retard ageing. Both areas are relatively new and it is difficult to speculate about their effects on long-term care needs, financing, and delivery. Nevertheless, while major breakthroughs resulting in increased life expectancy and improved health status of the elderly may reduce health and long-term care expenditures, they may also result in significant increases in pension and other social support service payments.

Conclusions

Over the last decade budget pressures in particular have led governments to become increasingly concerned with value for money. Much of the policy emphasis has shifted from access to efficiency. There is increasing evidence that the significant differences both within and across countries in spending and utilisation and intensity of services cannot be fully justified on the basis of quality and health outcomes. There is a growing body of evidence that indicates a widespread inappropriate use of hospitals and certain surgical and other diagnostic services. If the 18-day OECD average length of stay were to be reduced by just 1 day, savings in excess of $17 billion per year could be achieved. Similarly, only 80 per cent on average of inpatient beds are occupied at any given time. If half of this excess capacity could be eliminated (e.g. 10 per cent of beds), over $30 billion could be saved annually.

While these examples are simplistic[16], they provide some rather obvious indications of possible waste and excess capacity. Less obviously, substantial savings could also be achieved through reimbursement reforms and the reduction of inappropriate admissions to hospitals. Other savings could occur through extensive use, where medically appropriate, of outpatient surgery, mental health clinics, nursing homes, home health care, and more effective technology evaluation and planning. Cost-sharing, if appropriately structured, could also result in savings without major adverse effects on health outcomes. In the longer run, programmes focusing on consumer education, prevention and lifestyles could yield important results.

Current reforms and future policy choices both involve governments, either directly as the principal supplier of resources and finance, or indirectly in terms of its regulatory power. There are a number of reasons for this influential role, which is likely to continue. In the first place, the highly publicised successes of modern medicine over the past 40 years have conditioned the public to expect a technical solution to each and every perceived health care problem. Over a very wide range of illnesses, this expectation has been warranted. High and increasing success rates have encouraged patients to accept nothing less than a successful outcome. In those areas where it is known that technical "cures" do not yet exist, it has become difficult to admit that, given sufficient time and resources, one cannot be found. Such an attitude has not been discouraged, whether by consumers, practitioners, researchers or financing entities. Nevertheless, in the context of these current expectations, technological developments and changing population composition are forcing governments to make difficult decisions concerning the financing of health services and the rationing of certain technologies.

Second, pressure for government involvement persists because the provision of health care is regarded as a social good. The financing of health care services is a collective activity and its provision, in almost all countries, is assured by the State. This arises not only because of the need to provide insurance against catastrophic risk, but also because the provision of health care has become increasingly part of an inter-generational transfer from the working to the retired population whose health needs become greater as they age. Added to this task of providing general social insurance is the explicit desire on the part of all OECD countries to ensure universal coverage and equality of access.

Third, and in association with the expanding technology, it is clear that strong economic forces are involved. As preceding chapters have shown, communities are generally willing to devote an increasing proportion of their rising income to the consumption of health care services. The public appears to be generally satisfied with their health systems and happy to see their continued expansion. But policy-makers are concerned about the extent to which either this growth, or the satisfaction with it, reflects the open-ended way in which health care is financed, the pressures exerted by supplying professionals, or a lack of cost-consciousness on the part of the consumers and providers.

Finally, in those areas of health care systems where private provision and market incentives play a significant role, governments have not been willing to leave the outcome to the completely free play of market forces. For competition to work a certain amount of government oversight is required. The consumer is, to a considerable extent, protected from the consequences of his or her ignorance, minimum quality assurance is prescribed, and reimbursement rates for suppliers approximating some concept of efficient delivery are established.

Together these influences add up to a large and growing demand to which governments and policy-makers must respond. But in spite of the developments which are now taking place in the management of health systems, there are difficulties. As previous discussion has indicated, health outcomes and their responsiveness to changes in policy or expenditure are difficult to assess in either individual or collective terms. Many of the benefits of modern medicine cannot be quantified in terms of money, life expectancy or other social, medical or economic terms. There is also a growing ethical element in the decisions which must be taken. Reductions in pain and suffering, in premature deaths and in deformities, together with an increased capacity for work, leisure and enjoyment have all contributed to a high standard of living and an improved quality of life. Modern medicine has bestowed tremendous benefits on society. But the exigencies of budgets force policy-makers to interpret the value which society wishes to place on these considerable but often intangible benefits, and to weigh their priority relative to other, alternative, community goals.

Thus the central conclusion of this report is that both information and evaluation techniques fall short of what would be truly desirable for policy-making. There are ambiguities about evaluating what the public wants and what planners should be trying to achieve. There are major uncertainties about the way in which health systems and the people involved in them behave. Health outcomes are difficult to assess and the consequences of changes in policy or expenditure are even less well understood. And even though government decision-makers possess a fairly large armoury of policy instruments, little is known about their effectiveness in achieving overall social policy goals. In such circumstances both the formulation and the critique of policy are problematic.

Despite this apparently unsatisfactory picture concerning the underlying knowledge base and policy-making, there have been and continue to be significant advances. Governments no longer adopt simplistically the adage "more is better". Researchers and policy-makers are focusing their efforts on measuring outcomes, evaluating appropriateness of care, identifying vulnerable groups, basing policy changes implicitly or explicitly on outcome, equity, and economic efficiency criteria. Medical care providers are becoming increasingly aware of the cost consequences of their actions. New technologies are being evaluated in terms of medical and cost-effectiveness, as well as ethical considerations. Consumers are being educated in terms both of having more reasonable expectations and about the importance of lifestyles and prevention. The concept of limits is gradually being accepted by all the social partners. Thus, while governments may not (and indeed may never) have all the information they would like to have, they are aware of the problems and gaps. International collaboration and flows of information are increasing.

Many of these manifestations of health care financing, delivery, utilisation, and policy formulation have been magnified by the growing importance of the health sector. This importance has been due in large measure to the successes of health care financing programmes in promoting access and delivery systems capacity, as well as to the technical successes of modern medicine. While rapid growth in spending has been one result, so have increased life expectancy, reductions in premature deaths, and almost universal access to care. Yet these very successes have highlighted the difficult financial and ethical questions that all societies now face. Better evaluative tools and emphases on cost and medical effectiveness are the necessary concomitants to the consolidation of past gains and the accommodation of future changes.

NOTES AND REFERENCES

1. See J.W. Hurst, "The Scope for Developing Operational Measures of Health Outcome in the Next 5-10 Years", U.K. Department of Health and Social Security, London, 1985, pp. 1-2; and Walsh McDermott, "Absence of Indicators of the Influence of Its Physicians on a Society's Health", *The American Journal of Medicine*, Vol. 70, April 1981. Legislation was introduced in the United States Senate in early 1986 to establish a programme to evaluate the efficacy and quality of medical and surgical procedures in the $80 billion U.S. Medicare programme.

2. See for example, J.W. Hurst, *Financing Health Services in the United States, Canada and Britain*, Kind Edward's Hospital Fund, London, 1985, pp. 97-99.

3. See R. Illsley and P.-G. Svensson, *The Health Burden of Social Inequities*, World Health Organisation, Regional Office for Europe, Copenhagen, 1986; and Z.J. Brzezinski, *Mortality in the European Region*, World Health Organisation, Regional Office for Europe, Copenhagen, 1985.

4. See *Social Expenditure 1960-1990: Problems of Growth and Control*, OECD, Paris, 1985; Peter S. Heller, Richard Hemming and Peter W. Kohnert, *Ageing and Social Expenditure in the Major Industrialised Countries, 1980-2025*, Occasional Paper 47, International Monetary Fund, Washington, D.C., September 1986; *Reforming Public Pensions: Background, Pressures and Options*, OECD, Paris, forthcoming; and *The Social Policy Implications of Ageing Populations*, OECD, Paris, forthcoming.

5. For reviews of recent policy measures see "Recent Innovations in Social Policy: Secretariat Overview of National Reports", Internal Working Paper, OECD, Paris, 1985; *Report on the Committee for the Survey of Hospital and Nursing Home Trends and Planning*, Meeting No. 3, Association Internationale de la Mutualité, Geneva, June 7, 1985; *Report of the 15th General Assembly*, Association Internationale de la Mutualité, Geneva, September 1984; *Document Resulting from the Work of the Committee for the Survey of Relations With the Medical Profession*, Association Internationale de la Mutualité, Geneva, September 1984; *Measures Taken to Contain the Cost of Health in Europe*, Comité Europeen des Assurances, Paris, June 1985; and *National Commentaries 1984*, International Federation of Voluntary Health Service Funds, London, 1984.

6. See *Medicare Prospective Payment and the American Health Care System: Report to the Congress*, Prospective Payment Assessment Commission, Washington D.C., February 1986; and *Impact of the Medicare Hospital Prospective Payment System: 1984 Annual Report*, United States Department of Health and Human Services, Health Care Financing Administration, Baltimore, Maryland, August 1986.

7. Ira Burney and George J. Schieber, "Medicare Physicians' Services: The Composition of Spending and Assignment Rates", *Health Care Financing Review*, Fall 1985, pp. 91-92.

8. See A. Brandt, B. Horisberger and W.P. von Wartburg (eds.), *Cost Sharing in Health Care*, Springer-Verlag, Berlin, 1980; Wynand P.M.M. van de Ven, "Effects of Cost-Sharing in Health Care", *Effective Health Care*, June 1983; Robert H. Brook et al., *The Effect of Coinsurance on the Health of Adults*, Rand, Santa Monica, California, December 1984; and "Use of Medical Care in the Rand Health Insurance Experiment: Diagnosis- and Service-Specific Analyses in a Randomised Controlled Trial", *Medical Care*, Supplement, Vol. 24, No. 9, September 1986.

9. Emmett B. Keeler and John E. Rolph, "How Cost Sharing Reduced Medical Spending of Participants in the Health Insurance Experiment", *Journal of the American Medical Association*, Vol. 249, No. 16, April 22, 1983.

10. Kevin F. O'Grady et al., *The Impact of Cost Sharing on Emergency Department Use*, Rand, Santa Monica, California, October 1985.

11. Emmett B. Keeler et al., "How Free Care Reduced Hypertension in the Health Insurance Experiment", *Journal of the American Medical Association*, Vol. 254, No. 14, October 11, 1985.

12. It should be kept in mind that the Rand Experiment did not include any elderly individuals.

13. See Harold S. Luft, *Health Maintenance Organisations: Dimensions of Performance*, John Wiley and Sons, New York, 1981 and the updated version published by Transaction Books, New Brunswick, New Jersey, 1987; Julie Kosterlitz, "The Government Health Experts, Wall Street Pinning Their Hopes on HMOs", *National Journal*, Nov. 23, 1985; and Joseph P. Newhouse *et al.*, *Are Fee-for-Service Costs Increasing Faster Than HMO Costs*, Rand, Santa Monica, California, October 1985.

14. Harold S. Luft, "Introduction", *Health Maintenance Organisations: Dimensions of Performance* (1987), *Ibid*; and Harold S. Luft, "Alternative Delivery Systems: Applicability of the United States Experience With Health Maintenance Organisations to Other Countries", Internal Working Paper, OECD, Paris, 1987.

15. See *Long-Term Care for the Elderly Provided Within the Framework of Health Care Schemes*, International Social Security Association, XXIInd General Assembly, Montreal, 2-12 September, 1986, pp. 16-17.

16. They assume that marginal and average costs are the same, that proportionate reductions can take place across all countries, that other services are not substituted, and ignore the problem of geographic imbalances. Furthermore, it has been shown that significant savings occur when entire units or hospitals rather than individual beds are closed. Moreover, the stark political realities of trying to close excess facilities are well known.

OECD SALES AGENTS
DÉPOSITAIRES DES PUBLICATIONS DE L'OCDE

ARGENTINA - ARGENTINE
Carlos Hirsch S.R.L.,
Florida 165, 4º Piso,
(Galeria Guemes) 1333 Buenos Aires
Tel. 33.1787.2391 y 30.7122

AUSTRALIA-AUSTRALIE
D.A. Book (Aust.) Pty. Ltd.
11-13 Station Street (P.O. Box 163)
Mitcham, Vic. 3132   Tel. (03) 873 4411

AUSTRIA - AUTRICHE
OECD Publications and Information Centre,
4 Simrockstrasse,
5300 Bonn (Germany)   Tel. (0228) 21.60.45
Local Agent:
Gerold & Co., Graben 31, Wien 1 Tel. 52.22.35

BELGIUM - BELGIQUE
Jean de Lannoy, Service Publications OCDE,
avenue du Roi 202
B-1060 Bruxelles   Tel. (02) 538.51.69

CANADA
Renouf Publishing Company Ltd/
Éditions Renouf Ltée,
1294 Algoma Road, Ottawa, Ont. K1B 3W8
Tel: (613) 741-4333
Toll Free/Sans Frais:
Ontario, Quebec, Maritimes:
1-800-267-1805
Western Canada, Newfoundland:
1-800-267-1826
Stores/Magasins:
61 rue Sparks St., Ottawa, Ont. K1P 5A6
Tel: (613) 238-8985
211 rue Yonge St., Toronto, Ont. M5B 1M4
Tel: (416) 363-3171
Sales Office/Bureau des Ventes:
7575 Trans Canada Hwy, Suite 305,
St. Laurent, Quebec H4T 1V6
Tel: (514) 335-9274

DENMARK - DANEMARK
Munksgaard Export and Subscription Service
35, Nørre Søgade, DK-1370 København K
Tel. +45.1.12.85.70

FINLAND - FINLANDE
Akateeminen Kirjakauppa,
Keskuskatu 1, 00100 Helsinki 10   Tel. 0.12141

FRANCE
OCDE/OECD
Mail Orders/Commandes par correspondance :
2, rue André-Pascal,
75775 Paris Cedex 16
Tel. (1) 45.24.82.00
Bookshop/Librairie : 33, rue Octave-Feuillet
75016 Paris
Tel. (1) 45.24.81.67 or/ou (1) 45.24.81.81
Principal correspondant :
Librairie de l'Université,
12a, rue Nazareth,
13602 Aix-en-Provence   Tel. 42.26.18.08

GERMANY - ALLEMAGNE
OECD Publications and Information Centre,
4 Simrockstrasse,
5300 Bonn   Tel. (0228) 21.60.45

GREECE - GRÈCE
Librairie Kauffmann,
28, rue du Stade, 105 64 Athens Tel. 322.21.60

HONG KONG
Government Information Services,
Publications (Sales) Office,
Beaconsfield House, 4/F.,
Queen's Road Central

ICELAND - ISLANDE
Snæbjörn Jónsson & Co., h.f.,
Hafnarstræti 4 & 9,
P.O.B. 1131 – Reykjavik
Tel. 13133/14281/11936

INDIA - INDE
Oxford Book and Stationery Co.,
Scindia House, New Delhi 1 Tel. 331.5896/5308
17 Park St., Calcutta 700016   Tel. 240832

INDONESIA - INDONÉSIE
Pdii-Lipi, P.O. Box 3065/JKT.Jakarta
Tel. 583467

IRELAND - IRLANDE
TDC Publishers - Library Suppliers,
12 North Frederick Street, Dublin 1.
Tel. 744835-749677

ITALY - ITALIE
Libreria Commissionaria Sansoni,
Via Lamarmora 45, 50121 Firenze
Tel. 579751/584468
Via Bartolini 29, 20155 Milano Tel. 365083
Sub-depositari :
Editrice e Libreria Herder,
Piazza Montecitorio 120, 00186 Roma
Tel. 6794628
Libreria Hœpli,
Via Hœpli 5, 20121 Milano   Tel. 865446
Libreria Scientifica
Dott. Lucio de Biasio "Aeiou"
Via Meravigli 16, 20123 Milano   Tel. 807679
Libreria Lattes,
Via Garibaldi 3, 10122 Torino   Tel. 519274
La diffusione delle edizioni OCSE è inoltre
assicurata dalle migliori librerie nelle città più
importanti.

JAPAN - JAPON
OECD Publications and Information Centre,
Landic Akasaka Bldg., 2-3-4 Akasaka,
Minato-ku, Tokyo 107   Tel. 586.2016

KOREA - CORÉE
Kyobo Book Centre Co. Ltd.
P.O.Box: Kwang Hwa Moon 1658,
Seoul   Tel. (REP) 730.78.91

LEBANON - LIBAN
Documenta Scientifica/Redico,
Edison Building, Bliss St.,
P.O.B. 5641, Beirut   Tel. 354429-344425

MALAYSIA - MALAISIE
University of Malaya Co-operative Bookshop
Ltd.,
P.O.Box 1127, Jalan Pantai Baru,
Kuala Lumpur   Tel. 577701/577072

NETHERLANDS - PAYS-BAS
Staatsuitgeverij
Chr. Plantijnstraat, 2 Postbus 20014
2500 EA S-Gravenhage   Tel. 070-789911
Voor bestellingen: Tel. 070-789880

NEW ZEALAND - NOUVELLE-ZÉLANDE
Government Printing Office Bookshops:
Auckland: Retail Bookshop, 25 Rutland Street,
Mail Orders, 85 Beach Road
Private Bag C.P.O.
Hamilton: Retail: Ward Street,
Mail Orders, P.O. Box 857
Wellington: Retail, Mulgrave Street, (Head
Office)
Cubacade World Trade Centre,
Mail Orders, Private Bag
Christchurch: Retail, 159 Hereford Street,
Mail Orders, Private Bag
Dunedin: Retail, Princes Street,
Mail Orders, P.O. Box 1104

NORWAY - NORVÈGE
Tanum-Karl Johan
Karl Johans gate 43, Oslo 1
PB 1177 Sentrum, 0107 Oslo 1Tel. (02) 42.93.10

PAKISTAN
Mirza Book Agency
65 Shahrah Quaid-E-Azam, Lahore 3 Tel. 66839

PORTUGAL
Livraria Portugal,
Rua do Carmo 70-74, 1117 Lisboa Codex.
Tel. 360582/3

SINGAPORE - SINGAPOUR
Information Publications Pte Ltd
Pei-Fu Industrial Building,
24 New Industrial Road No. 02-06
Singapore 1953   Tel. 2831786, 2831798

SPAIN - ESPAGNE
Mundi-Prensa Libros, S.A.,
Castelló 37, Apartado 1223, Madrid-28001
Tel. 431.33.99
Libreria Bosch, Ronda Universidad 11,
Barcelona 7   Tel. 317.53.08/317.53.58

SWEDEN - SUÈDE
AB CE Fritzes Kungl. Hovbokhandel,
Box 16356, S 103 27 STH,
Regeringsgatan 12,
DS Stockholm   Tel. (08) 23.89.00
Subscription Agency/Abonnements:
Wennergren-Williams AB,
Box 30004, S104 25 Stockholm.
Tel. (08)54.12.00

SWITZERLAND - SUISSE
OECD Publications and Information Centre,
4 Simrockstrasse,
5300 Bonn (Germany)   Tel. (0228) 21.60.45
Local Agent:
Librairie Payot,
6 rue Grenus, 1211 Genève 11
Tel. (022) 31.89.50

TAIWAN - FORMOSE
Good Faith Worldwide Int'l Co., Ltd.
9th floor, No. 118, Sec.2
Chung Hsiao E. Road
Taipei   Tel. 391.7396/391.7397

THAILAND - THAILANDE
Suksit Siam Co., Ltd.,
1715 Rama IV Rd.,
Samyam Bangkok 5   Tel. 2511630

TURKEY - TURQUIE
Kültur Yayinlari Is-Türk Ltd. Sti.
Atatürk Bulvari No: 191/Kat. 21
Kavaklidere/Ankara   Tel. 25.07.60
Dolmabahce Cad. No: 29
Besiktas/Istanbul   Tel. 160.71.88

UNITED KINGDOM - ROYAUME-UNI
H.M. Stationery Office,
Postal orders only: (01)211-5656
P.O.B. 276, London SW8 5DT
Telephone orders: (01) 622.3316, or
Personal callers:
49 High Holborn, London WC1V 6HB
Branches at: Belfast, Birmingham,
Bristol, Edinburgh, Manchester

UNITED STATES - ÉTATS-UNIS
OECD Publications and Information Centre,
2001 L Street, N.W., Suite 700,
Washington, D.C. 20036 - 4095
Tel. (202) 785.6323

VENEZUELA
Libreria del Este,
Avda F. Miranda 52, Aptdo. 60337,
Edificio Galipan, Caracas 106
Tel. 32.23.01/33.26.04/31.58.38

YUGOSLAVIA - YOUGOSLAVIE
Jugoslovenska Knjiga, Knez Mihajlova 2,
P.O.B. 36, Beograd   Tel. 621.992

Orders and inquiries from countries where Sales
Agents have not yet been appointed should be sent
to:
OECD, Publications Service, Sales and
Distribution Division, 2, rue André-Pascal, 75775
PARIS CEDEX 16.

Les commandes provenant de pays où l'OCDE n'a
pas encore désigné de dépositaire peuvent être
adressées à :
OCDE, Service des Publications. Division des
Ventes et Distribution. 2. rue André-Pascal. 75775
PARIS CEDEX 16.

70712-04-1987

OECD PUBLICATIONS, 2, rue André-Pascal, 75775 PARIS CEDEX 16 - No. 43961 1987
PRINTED IN FRANCE
(81 87 02 1) ISBN 92-64-12973-1